Walt F.J. Goodridge, author of •*The Man Who Lived Forever* and • *Fit to Breed* and publisher of • *Fast & Grow Young* and •*The Power of Positive Eating After the Fast* presents:

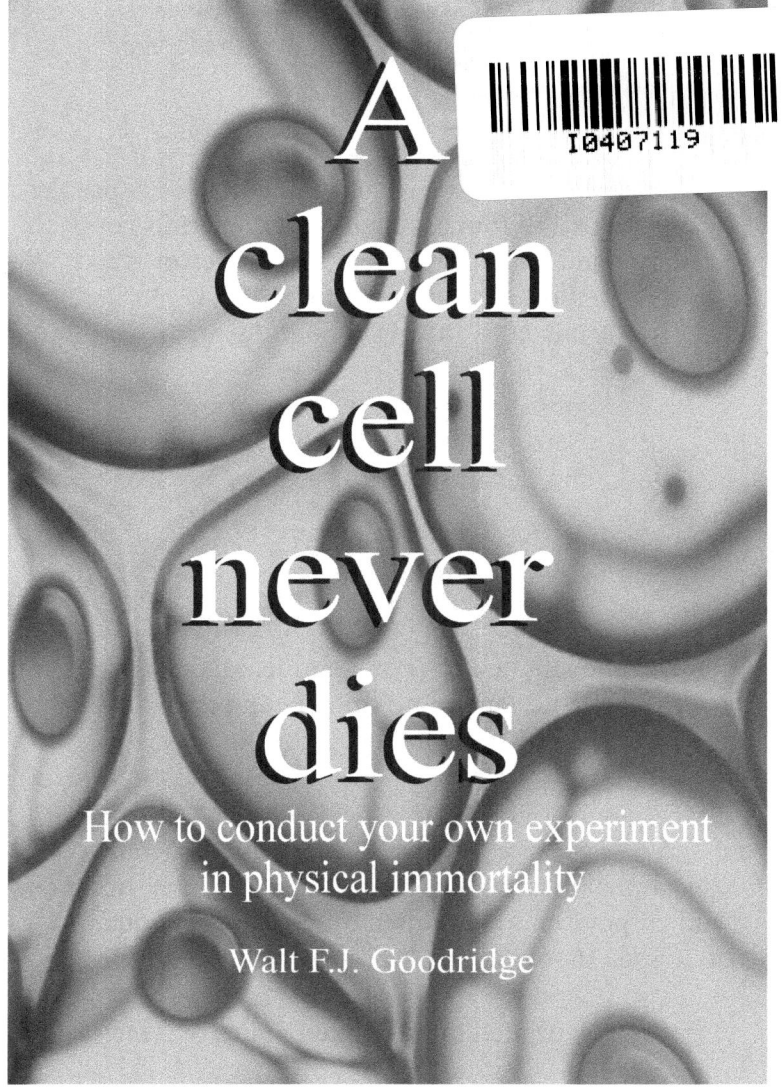

A clean cell never dies

How to conduct your own experiment in physical immortality

Walt F.J. Goodridge

A Clean Cell Never Dies
How to Conduct Your Own Experiment
in Physical Immortality
(Volume 3 in the Ageless Adept™ Series)
© Walt F.J. Goodridge. All rights reserved.

ISBN-13: 9781540755414

Published by Walt F.J. Goodridge
dba a company called W
dba The Passion Profit Company

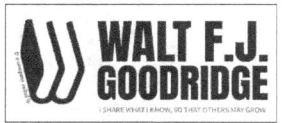

Books, coaching, apps, audio, video, merchandise,
courses, freebies and more from a company called W!
www.waltgoodridge.com

Cover image of cells by: Zoya Fedorova (123rf.com)

Educational institutions, government agencies, libraries
and corporations are invited to inquire about quantity
discounts. (646) 481-4238 | sales@waltgoodridge.com

Paperback printed in the United States of America

Table of Contents

Dedication ▲
This book is dedicated to the extremists

Acknowledgments ▲
Thanks to Lisa Hacskaylo for her assistance in communicating with the non-extremists!

A Necessary Disclaimer ▲

For legal reasons based on the prevailing societal paradigm, I must include the following:

The purpose of this guide is to provide my experiences and observations. It is for anyone who wants to learn about my experiences. I am not a doctor, and do not claim to be one.

The information in this guide is not intended to be a substitute for professional advice. It is only meant to complement, not replace any advice or information from a "health professional." You should not use this information to diagnose or treat health problems or disease without consulting a qualified "health care provider" with any questions or concerns you may have regarding your condition, or ways in which to use alternative therapies. I, the author of this book, disclaim any personal liability or loss caused or alleged to be caused, through application of the information in this guide.

As a result of each person's unique lifestyle, choices, history, exposure, path and inherited traits, each person's body has arrived at a unique place in its development, rejuvenation and/or deterioration and will, therefore, react differently, even to natural substances. As much as this guide contains merely suggestions of natural substances and natural practices, if you are currently on pharmaceutical medication of any kind, then your body's system is most likely compromised, and even natural foods could have an adverse effect on you.

Any strategy you implement must, therefore, be administered on an individual basis, and it would be wise to consult a holistic healing practitioner familiar with the contraindications of real food when combined with unnatural drugs and chemicals that may be present in your body.

The content herein is not intended to diagnose or prescribe treatment for any illness. Use them as informational only.

"In a world based on lies,
the truth is considered subversive"

Preliminary ▲

How to Use This Book

(a) To get the most from this book, never continue reading past a word or phrase you don't understand! It's been shown that the only reason people give up on a new project or course of study is that they encounter a word, phrase or concept for which they have no definition, or the wrong definition. If a word in this guide is new to you, please use a dictionary to find the most accurate definition. This is important.

(b) Investigate each item. This is not an encyclopedia. It's a guidebook--a road map with an available route, destination and a checklist of milestones along the way. Take the time to fully explore each suggestion to really optimize the journey! (c) Read it at least twice—once for a general overview, and again and again as you take action!

My Position

"I am not here to convince, justify, defend or apologize for my beliefs, choices or lifestyle. I'm not here for validation, vindication or approval, or to respond to personal attacks. I'm here to share a philosophy and formula that work for me and for others. In a world of seven billion people, if one person can do a thing, then it must be possible for at least one other person to do the same. It is against this backdrop that I wrote this book."

Steps of the Scientific Method

The main steps scientists take when conducting scientific inquiry on a given subject are:

1. Make an observation
2. Form a question
3. State a hypothesis
4. Conduct an experiment
5. Analyze the data and draw a conclusion

Applied to *A Clean Cell Never Dies*:

1. Make an observation.

I learned that a doctor once kept cells alive for over 20 years by providing nutrients and removing waste. I've noticed that because of my lifestyle and some of my dietary practices to supply my body with proper nutrients and keep the cells of my body clean that I am not showing the typical signs of accumulated years in the same way my friends and relatives are.

2. Form a question.

What would happen if a person practiced this diet and these behaviors in a methodical and consistent way with the express goal of longevity?

3. Form a hypothesis

A hypothesis is an informed guess as to the possible answer to the question. The purpose of the hypothesis is not to arrive at the perfect answer to the question but to provide a direction to further scientific investigation.

I hypothesize, based on Carrel's experiment, that a person who adequately nourishes and removes waste from the cells of the body can, if not survive indefinitely, suspend or delay the aging process.

4. Conduct an experiment.

This book shall provide the reader with direction for further investigation and experimentation. While this book neither claims nor desires to meet the standard criteria for a "scientific" experiment, all the evidence and elements needed to deduce certain truths about the world are already at your disposal. No double-blind, placebo-controlled study necessary. Nature is your laboratory. Your body is your subject. Your state of health on your previous lifestyle (and, quite frankly, the rest of the world) is your control group. Our experiment is definitely "reproducible" as all of the suggestions are within most people's ability to achieve and practice.

5. Analyze the data and draw a conclusion.

The reader is encouraged to note the findings of the experiment for personal benefit as well as for others who may follow in these footsteps.

About this book

IMPORTANT: Please do not skim through these introductory sections as people—even myself—often do. You see, if you are constantly sick or prematurely aging, it's because something about your underlying belief system as it relates to health and wellness is out of alignment with truth. Therefore, in order to help you overcome these beliefs, you need to understand the foundational basis and philosophy behind this book. It is all very, very necessary. Please indulge me, therefore, and don't simply rush to the good parts. In fact, it might be that very rush to immediate gratification that is contributing to your premature aging, so here is where you can start to execute the Clean Cell secret by doing things a little differently! A few years ago, I wrote *The Ageless Adept*, now known as *The Man Who Lived Forever*. It is the tale of one man's search for, introduction to and implementation of a set of beliefs, practices and lifestyle for perfect health, long life and the fountain of youth. It contains all the underlying beliefs, philosophy, mindset and worldview I practice and preach in regard to health, wellness and rejuvenation. This book, however, (*A Clean Cell Never Dies*), expands upon that work with the answer to "How exactly do you stay so young-looking?" It contains:

My personal experience

Many authors create books based on conventional wisdom, studies and third party information. I never recommend anything I've not personally tried.

A promise that THIS IS REAL!

Yes, age reversal through Clean Cell living is possible. I doubted it myself, because even though I was able to achieve results personally, I wasn't sure if I could help others do the same. Now that I'm it with others, it has become clear that, combined with the right mindset and understanding, it can absolutely, positively produce results and help you peel back the pages of the calendar!

This is neither speculation nor conjecture. This is not fiction. What I wish to impart to you is that, despite what you may believe about aging, retaining youthfulness, physical energy and stamina, it doesn't have to be that way. It is possible to slip through the hands of time. That's my promise to you.

Why I wrote this book

I compiled and wrote the information in this book because I want to keep my friends and family around for a long time, too. It's simply no fun to watch people deteriorating due to what is often simply a lack of information. I want everyone to enjoy the same excitement for life and have the desire and energy as I do to bound out of bed each day and enjoy that life. I want my girlfriends to enjoy my own as well as their own bodies' capacities for pleasure. And, as more and more people ask me about my health practices, I want to share what I know to a wider audience.

Who this book is for

"In our society, we've been sold a childish belief that we can continue our destructive behaviors, yet expect to reap creative benefits. We want to taste the sugar, but not experience its effects. We want to live in excess, without the accumulation. We then place our hopes in magic pills or potions that will wipe away the effects of our actions."— *The Man Who Lived Forever*

As an independent author with a passion for sharing what I know, I write to share my truth-- nontraditional as it may be branded. The challenge is that in our society, there is an inordinate amount of emphasis placed on immediate gratification, comfort and ease. We are led to believe we should only eat things that taste good, engage in activities that feel good, and avoid any and all discomfort at all costs.

You see, through no fault of our own (or, more accurately, through no choice we remember), we've ended up on a planet where deception and insanity are the orders of the day, if not the rule of law. We "celebrate" our good fortune by poisoning ourselves with alcohol and sugar. Businesses are allowed to sell cancer-causing chemicals and call it food. We kill, skin, burn, bake and consume the bodies of other creatures and call it fine dining. This paradigm was never conceived of nor developed in order to support our health, well being and happiness. Other authors may attempt to show you how to survive within it. I, on the other hand, subversively advocate its overthrow! The paradigm is what is killing you!

Consequently, although written with the intention of helping as many people as possible, this book is unlikely to reach beyond a much narrower range. Why? One premise of this book is that if you wish to take control of your health, live longer and healthier and reverse the aging process, you can either (a) find the courage and discipline to live outside the current paradigm of beliefs and behavior, or (b) resolve to accept your fate and stop whining about the decline.

"There can be no success without discipline."

This book offers no magic pill, no fairy dust and no silver bullet path to health. The only way to reverse the effects of a lifetime of poor choices is to retrain yourself to make different and better choices until those new choices become the norm. And given what passes as "the norm" in our society, such a decision will require discipline.

This book is not--to paraphrase the title of a popular book from the 1970s--*The Lazy Man's Way to Health & Wellness*. The concept of discipline, delay and deprivation as necessary for health isn't easily digested by a population programmed since birth to seek comfort and ease. This book is for a small group of folks willing to approach life differently, and willing to do the necessary work to achieve the desired outcome. This book is for the extremists. To paraphrase Senator Barry Goldwater's speech writer Karl Hess' use of an idea with its origins creditable to either Cicero or US President Lincoln:

*"Extremism in defense of health is not a vice.
Moderation in pursuit of immortality is no virtue."*

And for everyone else ready for change!

What if you don't feel you have that discipline? Don't worry, our society is evolving. People are awakening to the effects of factory farming, greenhouse gases, genetically-modified foods, climate change, pesticides, etc., and consequently, manufacturers, stores and even entire communities are responding. As historically long-lived "hotspots" around the world (think Okinawa's and the Mediterranean's longest-lived people) and the ground breaking Blue Zone Project® communities based on those societies have demonstrated, we can, and do make healthy choices when the places we live, work, learn, and play and spend 90% of our time (grocery stores, restaurants, work sites, schools, churches, playgrounds) are reshaped to support those choices.

This book, therefore, is for everyone else whose social groups and surroundings are already making it increasingly easier to live the Clean Cell lifestyle!

And who am I?

My name is Walt F.J. Goodridge. I'm the author of over 25 books including *Turn Your Passion Into Profit* and *Living True to Your Self* and their associated philosophies and formulas. I'm also a vegan, a bit of a health nut and, as "The Ageless Adept," am author of *Fit to Breed* and publisher of *Fast & Grow Young*. Regardless of the subject matter, my prime directive remains the same: to empower others with information, inspiration and ideas to help them reclaim their power, break free and live true to themselves!

Let's begin!

á-dept – *n*. 1. a person who is skilled or proficient at something. (note accent on the a); "they are adepts at kung fu and karate" synonyms: expert, master, genius, maestro, doyen, virtuoso

CHAPTER 1: Experiments ▲

"Perfect health, long life and eternal youth are not the random, genetic blessings of a chaotic or capricious universe, but natural birthrights that can be accessed through the mindful acceptance of simple truths, activated by the disciplined practice of proven activities, and sustained by advancement along a known path. This is that path."--The Ageless Adept

The Basis

On January 17, 1912, Nobel Prize winner Dr. Alexis Carrel began a famous experiment at the Rockefeller Institute for Medical Research in which he placed tissue cultured from an embryonic chicken heart in a flask of his own design. He maintained the living culture for well over 20 years--much longer than a chicken's normal life span--proving that living cells could be kept alive indefinitely by simply controlling the nutrients and removing the waste in the surrounding solution.

Proper nutrition and removal of waste. This is the simple formula for longevity for which no practical lifestyle guide has ever existed. Our failure practicing this formula is the cause of most, if not all, disease.

This book will show you how to fulfill those two simple requirements in practical ways to effectively conduct your own experiment in bodily immortality.

My experiment

One evening many years ago, I attended a college reunion about ten years after graduation. Towards the end of the evening, the host of the event invited questions and comments from the attendees. Wilton C., a former classmate of mine, raised his hand to ask a question.

"Here's what I'd like to know," Wilton began. "I want to know how come Walt looks younger *now*, than when he was here in college!?"

Although Wilton may have asked rhetorically and in jest, I felt compelled to give an answer. I had been vegan for about four years at the time, but I told him and everyone else that I believed it was that lifestyle—and the courage and discipline it required of me—that had everything to do with the answer he sought.

Friends and family, too, wonder how it is that I look younger now than when I was, um, "younger." I visited New York recently for a family gathering, and upon entering the room, the first question my aunts and uncle asked was if I dyed my hair. (The answer was and is 'no.') In addition, and for the record, my lovers are pleased with my youthful strength and stamina, but perhaps that's a bit too much information best reserved for another book. (See *Fit to Breed*)

However, it isn't simply being vegetarian that accounts for my immunity to the years and my success at reclaiming yesterday's me. Over those same years,

I've done quite a bit of reading and research, and have developed a set of my own "secret" practices based on my growing knowledge of supplements, herbs, food, vitamins, natural remedies and youth-retaining strategies.

I've personally used every one of the products and practices listed in this book. These secrets keep my hair black, my eyes bright, my skin glowing, my stomach flat and my energy level high. Yes, not only am I still alive, I am, in fact, healthier, younger looking, and more energetic than I was twenty years ago, and consider myself an over-achieving member of society with numerous published books, online businesses and a nomadpreneur lifestyle! These have been the results of *my* experiment.

In this book, I'm going to delve a little deeper into those practices and share the foods, herbs and other products you can obtain at a combination of neighborhood markets, health food stores, over the Internet and some you can even make yourself in your own home. You can use this information to conduct your own experiment.

Don't allow anyone to scare you away from this information!

Your experiment

I call this your experiment because that is exactly what it is. There are no double-blind, placebo controlled studies and research to back this up. You will be your own case study. You will be your own focus group. You are your own authority. There are, however, thousands of individual testimonials, anecdotal evidence, patient records of holistic practitioners, historical, cultural knowledge that attest to the effectiveness of each and every one of these suggested substances and practices. You can find them increasing in numbers on the Internet. Do your own research (be wary of the comments of those who seek to scare you). Then, once you've convinced yourself of the safety and harmlessness of the products and practices, and the sanity and soundness of the principles upon which their use is based, you will need to decide to embark on your own experiment.

I suggest that it should be the goal of your experiment to determine if these habits, practiced diligently, keep the cells of your body clean, youthful and rejuvenating. You may find, as I did, that they do!

CHAPTER 2: Foundation ▲

To be successful in any undertaking, it is first necessary to have the right paradigm.

Without the correct paradigm for your body and how it operates, for example, you will find that health eludes you despite your best efforts at eating healthy and living a healthy lifestyle.

Without the correct paradigm for health and how to achieve it, what you will find is that as you "cure" one ailment you will invariably create another.

Without the correct paradigm for Nature, you will find that you subvert the natural order, interfere with the ecological balance, destroy Nature's interconnectedness and create a host of other illnesses and imbalances within the body as well as environmentally

In order to provide those necessary paradigms, let's have a few conversations as orientation.

A New Foundation

There are two foundational ideas you'll need to accept and embrace to gain the most benefit from this and other books in the Ageless Adept™ series:

Idea one: You are your own authority

You don't need a PhD to understand your body, and you don't need anyone's permission to eat an apple. As eloquently spoken by author, Jerry Mander:

📖 [We must] make it easier for people to know about themselves, how they function, what a human being is, and how the human fits into the wider natural systems of the universe. This will make it possible for the human to recognize what is natural and real from what is artificial and contrived. People can achieve greater control of themselves, their needs, and their health, and find the answers they need on their own without the input of so-called experts and authorities from outside the self. Personal knowledge and experience is the best authority."

(Four Arguments for the Elimination of Television)

This is an important idea. You must dispense with the belief that someone else has more authority than you when it comes to what you put into your body. If this concept is daunting to you, this book may make it easier to believe and act upon this idea

Idea two: Everything you believe...is wrong

Before we can get to that place where we respect and embrace our own authority, we must first look at the world as objectively as possible. We must be willing to create a new belief system. This house of cards we refer to as society's current belief system is toppling. The cloak of deception upon which that system was based is unraveling. Everything we've been told, believe and accept as "true" about many aspects of reality is being challenged and exposed as simply false and wrong. Priests are being exposed as predators. Politicians are exposed as agenda-driven individualists rather than selfless public servants. Everything we believe is "progress" is unsustainable and propelling our planet towards extinction.

Everything you believe is "medicine" is often a set of untested drugs that unbalance the body's natural systems and cause more side effects than the illnesses they purport to cure.

Everything you believe is "food" are chemically laden substances that are unusable by the body, clog the system, deprive and rob the body of nutrients and its ability to heal itself.

Everything you believe is "economic growth through capitalism" is actually a money-grab that only benefits a select few at the expense of everyone else.

Everything you believe is "justice" is punitive, revenge-focused, violence-based thought and action that support a prison industry that enriches its owners.

Everything you've been told are the random events of history might actually have been orchestrated.

Everything you believe is "news" is sensationalized opinion, often completely contrived.

Everything you've been told to strive for in the pursuit of "success and freedom" actually lead to servitude and failure.

Everything you've been told, and thus believe is good, normal, necessary, desirable, ethical and moral are being revealed to be their exact opposites.

Everything you've been told and believe is evil, sinful, impossible, absurd and abnormal might actually be good, ethical, plausible, logical, quite normal and, in fact, might be in your best interest to explore.

The list goes on. Our beliefs about science, democracy, religion, government, education, the causes of war, the reasons behind assassinations, the existence of life on other planets, the origin of mankind, sexuality and various other concepts, ideas institutions and world views—are all being subjected to an onslaught of new questions, analyses and activism as people discover them to be other than what they've been led to believe is true.

When it comes to health, everything you believe about the body and how to maintain it--as well as illness and how to avoid it--is, quite simply, wrong.

This may come as a surprise, but it's entirely possible that everything you believe to be true about food, medicine, health, illness and aging is nothing more than a set of subjective ideas put forth by people who really don't have a handle on truth, don't know what they're doing, or worse, don't have your best interests at heart—people who are playing by a faulty rule book, or worse, with no rule book at all.

Uninformed ideas, blind assumptions and outright lies underlie many of the food and drug commercials on television and radio. I'm sure you're familiar with many of these assumptions: that milk does a body good; that meat is real food for real people; that cancer can't be cured; that the common cold is inevitable; that allergies can only be relieved not ended; that hormone levels, hair growth and one's virility and vitality inevitably decrease at certain ages; and that the drugs these companies are pushing heal and aren't, in fact, more dangerous than the ills they claim to cure, given the extensive list of (sometimes fatal) side effects warned of in the disclaimers.

The sales pitches for these products start with these assumptions as given and are never challenged. As a result, people buy into them (key word "buy"), and continue a vicious cycle perpetuating the very lifestyle that caused their ills.

Society seems to have lost a vital road map and is devolving in a direction that serves to support the industries that profit from peddling the products. These products allow people to believe they can maintain their destructive lifestyles, while purchasing so-called "cures" that, in actuality, do nothing more than temporarily relieve, mask or replace the symptoms of the illnesses the lifestyles cause.

If I believed, for example, that "milk does a body good," and acted on that belief (by drinking lots of milk) in an effort to improve my health, I might find myself experiencing colds, allergies, weakened bones and cancer, and eventually become frustrated in my efforts to achieve health without ever knowing the real reason why: that dairy products we've been told are beneficial, are, in fact poison to our systems!

For those pursuing a new paradigm of health, wellness, disease, aging and youth, what we need are:
• a lens of stable truths through which to see the world
• a new view of Nature that encourages new questions
• a method of critical analysis to arrive at new answers
• new possibilities and choices based on those answers
• a common sense philosophy on which to base lifestyle practices, built upon unchanging truths.

Let's begin that quest for a new set of stable truths. Stay with me! Remember, everything is necessary!

The 7 Truths of Reality

"In order to survive as a physical being
you must master the physical universe.
In order to master the physical universe,
you must know its truths."

The following 7 Truths are known and shared by mystics, philosophers, sages, seekers and adepts on all paths--essential knowledge that should be taught in every school, but are often hidden from the masses. *(Search online for "public domain Kybalion")*

Truth: The Truth of Mind
The first truth, the Truth of Mind, holds that all reality starts first as thought and belief. To achieve any desired end, therefore, you must first make yourself believe in the reality of what you wish to achieve. As it relates to this discussion, you must first believe it is possible and inevitable that you will reverse aging.

Truth: The Truth of Correspondence
Second is the Truth of Correspondence that states 'as above, so below.' What is truth above must be truth below. Stated still in another way, if a principle is true in matters of spirit, then it must be true in matters of flesh, otherwise it is not truth. If something claims to be truth but has conditions, contradictions, catches (or a whole bunch of side effects), it is most likely either a religion or an advertisement for a prescription drug!

Truth: The Truth of Motion
Third is the Truth of Motion that states that everything in the universe is in a state of motion. Everything vibrates. Every object, every action, every thought and every state of being is merely energy in a

unique state of vibration and motion. In other words, nothing is fixed or motionless or unchangeable—this is good to know when seeking to reverse aging.

Truth: The Truth of Duality

Fourth is the Truth of Duality that states that extremes of anything are just degrees of a single thing. In other words, *"...opposites are identical in nature, but different in degree."* For example, heat and cold are really the same thing (temperature) differing only in degree. Black and white, love and hate, east and west, and similarly, health and illness are extremes of one thing differing only by degree. The path of change, therefore, proceeds from one pole to the other. The path from illness to health (from aging to youthfulness) can be conceptualized as such.

Truth: The Truth of Rhythm

Fifth is the Truth of Rhythm that states that all things rise and fall. There is always action and reaction, back and forth, high tide and low tide, inflow and outflow in all things, including health.

Truth: The Truth of Cause and Effect

Sixth is the Truth of Cause and Effect that states nothing is random. Everything you experience is the direct result of some cause. Your thoughts are first cause, your actions are the means, and the conditions of your body are the effects. Despite common belief, health is not mysterious, and illness is not random. Both proceed by the law of cause and effect. You experience either to the degree you create it. You are always "at cause" for your health.

Truth: The Truth of Gender

Seventh is the Truth of Gender that states there is masculine and feminine in all things. Whether on a physical, mental or spiritual plane, the principles of father/mother, God/Nature, seed/womb are always in operation. Creation, generation, regeneration and the secret to creating youthfulness, all rely on this truth.

These truths comprise the totality of every phenomenon we know to exist and those we don't. Everything in the universe is based on these simple, stable truths. If the universe were not based on reliable, predictable truths, everything would collapse.

Two truths in particular, the Truth of Duality (everything is one thing and therefore reversible), and the Truth of Cause and Effect (nothing is random), are particularly important to our discussion of health.

The Seven Conversations

These conversations are based on 7 truths. Their goal is to empower you to be your own authority. It is essential to understand and accept the principle of the *first* conversation in order for them all to make sense.

1. Nature is foolproof.
2. The body is coded to heal.
3. There is only one disease.
4. There is only one cure.
5. Food and fasting facilitate flow.
6. There is one hindrance to health.
7. There is one challenge to change.

The full versions appear in *The Man Who Lived Forever.* However, I'll summarize them here.

Conversation 1: Nature is foolproof

Nature, as an entity, survives via the survival of its individual components—plants, animals, oceans, ecosystems etc. The activities of survival are simple enough so one does not need higher degrees to grasp or execute them: Predators seek prey. Animals mate by instinct. Seeds grow by design. Bees pollinate flowers. Animals seek brightly colored fruit. Everything proceeds seamlessly in ways that are foolproof (i.e., even a fool couldn't screw them up!)

In *The Man Who Lived Forever*, the adept questions the seeker about Nature and God*:

"Seeker, if you were God*, perfect, wise and omnipotent—would you create a world and a system of survival that required Ph.Ds to master? Or would you make it foolproof, so that even the least of your creations could negotiate it?"

"I guess I'd make it simple," I replied.

"And the truth is, Seeker, it is simple. God is not complicated. Complex, vast, infinite, perhaps, but not complicated. Nature is a simple, closed, self-contained system coded for survival. In other words, everything Nature needs for its own survival is already built right in. It's a 'batteries included' universe, if you will."

Conversation 2: The body is coded to heal

As an individual unit of Nature, your body is coded for healing, reversal, regeneration, renewal and rejuvenation. Cuts heal. Broken bones mend. Fevers kill germs. Yes, provided with the raw materials it needs, and left to its own intelligence, the body is designed to heal, survive, and thrive. Everything you currently define as illness is actually healing taking place. Diarrhea, colds and coughs, for instance, are all efforts by your body to cleanse and heal itself.

Note: age reversal using the clean cell practices does not require belief in a deity. Universal order exists for all

We're even told by experts that the body's organs renew themselves regularly, and that the entire body is completely renewed every seven years.

You might ask, "If the body is coded to heal, why am I and everyone I know deteriorating?" You'll answer that question by the time you finish this book. First, we'll explore how the body deteriorates.

Conversation 3: There is only one illness

Arnold Ehret, Charlotte Gerson and other healers have all shown and stated in their own ways that there is only one illness. (Remember, everything is one thing.) Un-reversed, this one illness starts to manifest in different parts of the body. Here are some common conditions along with explanations of how each is a manifestation of a single "disease."

Body odor: Unnatural substances accumulate and rot within your colon, putrefy, decay and spread to your body's tissues and organs, and then cause odors to emanate from your glands, feces and sweat.

Colds: A cold is the body's attempt to purge foreign elements--the body's effort to rid itself of accumulation. As your body's immune system gets more compromised by congestion, it gets less able to deal with invading pathogens and accumulated mucus. You don't "catch" a cold, you devolve into one.

Bad breath: Except for the odors caused by rotting teeth and infected gums (which are themselves the results of unnatural accumulation), "bad breath" comes from accumulations deeper within your digestive tract.

Backaches: Pounds of undigested matter can put pressure on the skeleton and muscles of the back; also caused by the localized accumulation of toxins.

Impotence: Clogged—constipated—blood vessels

limiting the flow of blood to extremities. Of course this can be caused by emotional blockage as well.

Depression--Mood-altering chemicals in the food upset your hormonal balance, and pollute the purity of the blood flow to the brain.

Multiple Sclerosis, Fibromyalgia, Chronic Fatigue and other chronic illness share common symptoms and causes. Accumulations of aspartame, depletion of magnesium and gold and chemical exposure have been cited as factors, that treated, have led to cures.

We could go on, but the only thing ever wrong with us is there's something *inside* the body that shouldn't be there, or something that *should* be there that isn't; an excess of the bad, or an absence of the good.

Therefore, regardless of the many names doctors may use, a single issue is at cause. Ehret calls it constipation. Gerson calls it toxicity. I call it blockage.

Blockage means there is (a) something inside the body that is being blocked from coming out, or (b) something outside the body blocked from coming in. There is something ingested or absorbed that stayed in, or something missing that must be assimilated. Illness is either an accumulation or a void of some kind.

Blockage (or constipation, or toxicity) occurs when things are introduced into the body that are not in harmony with its coding. We eat processed, refined, artificially flavored, colored, pasteurized, homogenized, fried, filtered and altered food, that is simply not natural. The body, which was never designed to handle these unnatural substances, suffers from accumulations and deposits and gets clogged. These clogs result in increased toxicity. The toxicity gets chronic (persisting for a long time), and deterioration results. The body's natural code is further suppressed, and more disease results.

Conversely, the flip side of blockage is depletion. We eat depleted foods and never adequately replenish the depletion of vitamins, minerals etc. the body requires for optimal function and to execute its healing code. The mystery is not why we get sick. The real mystery is how we stay alive given all the damage and depletion to which we subject ourselves.

Conversation 4: There is only one cure

If there is only one illness, it stands to reason there is only one cure. If blockage exists, the cure must be something that encourages the opposite of blockage. The opposite of blockage is flow.

When the pipes in your home are clogged and blocked, you call a plumber or use some other means to clean them out and restore the flow through the pipe. Similarly, when blockage occurs in our bodies, the cure is to introduce a flow.

Every illness caused by accumulation can be cured by release. Similarly, every illness that is the result of depletion can be cured by replenishment. But, we'll get to that later. A great percent of all blockage can be cured simply by allowing the body the time and resources it needs to return to a state of flow.

Your task, in order to stop the downward spiral, heal yourself, and reverse the aging process, is to adopt a lifestyle that respects and utilizes the healing and rejuvenating power of flow. This applies to all areas of your life, not just your diet. In other words:

Let your feelings flow. Releasing pent-up emotions is cathartic. It'll keep your heart young.

Let your clutter flow. Make room for the new by getting rid of the old, and you'll keep your environment young.

Let your money flow. Tithing, sharing, donating some of your wealth keeps abundance flowing and growing in your life and keeps your pockets young!

Let your talents—your passion—flow. Allowing yourself to be a channel for the flow of creation in this universe keeps your mind and spirit young. Yes, the secret to the Fountain of Youth is flow.

To determine how best to restore that flow in our bodies and in our lives, let's look to the natural environment and make some observations of truths and concepts you need to be aware of.

The Truth of Rhythm says where there is 'inflow' there must be 'outflow.' So if blockage (illness) implies a blockage of intake and output, then flow (cure) must imply a flow in as well as a flow out. Eating is inflow. Elimination is outflow. The two working together are the basis of health. As flow improves, health results. As flow becomes blockage, disease and illness result. According to the Truth of Rhythm, every "in" must have an "out." For every assimilation, there must be a corresponding elimination. The simple reason many people in this society are ill is because they never give their bodies the time or means to eliminate.

Flow is the key

To get the most from any engine, it's not the amount or even the quality of fuel that matters most, it's the efficiency of the engine! Two engines can use the same amount and quality of fuel—say one gallon of gas—and one engine will travel 23 miles, while the other, more efficient engine will travel 50!

Similarly, your performance is based on your body's efficiency. So, how does one create an efficient, vital human engine? Here's the formula adapted from *Arnold Ehret's Mucusless Diet & Healing System*:

The Vitality Formula is: $V = P^2 - O$

"V" is VITALITY.

"P^2" is POTENTIAL POWER, the available strength to keep you alive, drive the human machinery, and provide strength and endurance.

"O" is OBSTRUCTION, foreign matter, mucus, parasites, and anything that hinders circulation, the function of the organs, and flow. In other words,, blockage. In words, the formula is:

Vitality equals Potential Power minus Obstruction

Let's say you have 100 imaginary units of potential power (P^2) in your body, but you have 25 units of obstruction (O) in your colon. The amount of vitality your body has available to expend, therefore, is only 75.

$$100(P^2)ower - 25(O)bstruction = 75(V)itality$$

You can see by this equation that as soon as "O" becomes greater than "P" the human machine must come to a standstill. Yes, $V = P^2 - O$ is the formula of life and vitality, and at the same time you may call it the formula for illness and death.

Conversation 5: Food and fasting facilitate flow.

Eating real food and fasting for extended periods are two ways to facilitate flow in the body. More later.

Conversation 6: There is one hindrance to health.

The greatest hindrance to health in our modern society is the deception surrounding body, healing, wellness and disease.

Conversation 7: There is one challenge to change

The major challenge to change is finding the disciplined self. We touched on this earlier.

CHAPTER 3: Reversal ▲

What's really aging you

Before we talk about the concept of age reversal, let's discover what actually ages you.

Your belief system ages you

It's not simply time that ages you. The things you believe about the universe, the world, your environment, other people and yourself as well as your role and relationship to all of the above are all factors.

Your diet ages you

Of course, your diet plays a major role in the aging process. This book will focus on this.

Your habits age you

Your rate of "deterioration" is affected, not just by your eating habits, but habits related to sex, exercise, smoking, entertainment, etc.

Your environment ages you

Pollution, second-hand smoke, air conditioning, fluorescent lights, cell phone/tower radiation, laptops, microwaves and radon in the environment age you.

Your ability to remove waste ages you

There's a saying that "death begins in the colon." The condition of your colon and excretory organs (liver, kidney, skin) contribute to your rate of aging.

Toxic relationships age you

Some experts say every illness is a physical manifestation of an emotional or psychological issue and each of the body's organs correlates to a particular emotion. Fear manifests in the kidneys. Anxiety and sorrow in the lungs. Anger in the liver. Toxic relationships may be triggering illness and aging you as much as toxic food.

Your passionless existence ages you

Living a stressful life of working for survival, money and others' concepts of "success" with no outlet for the expression of your passions ages you.

Your predominant emotional state ages you

Most people view emotions as a hodge podge of moods and reactions that come and go, ebb and flow based on situation, circumstances or day of the week.

Although he wasn't the first, L. Ron Hubbard, author of *Dianetics*, presented some insightful research into the nature of human behavior and emotions which, he posited, fall within a distinct and ordered hierarchy called the tone scale.

As you move up the tone scale, life improves. As you move down the scale, life gets worse. Here is a chart representing the scale and the associated numeric values for each emotional state:

Emotional Survival (Tone) Scale

Serenity 40
Exhilaration 8.0
Enthusiasm 4.0
Cheerfulness 3.5
Strong Interest 3.3
Conservatism 3.0
Mild interest 2.9
Contentment 2.8
Disinterest 2.6
Boredom 2.5
Antagonism 2.0
Hostility 1.9
Pain 1.8
Anger 1.5
Hate 1.4
Resentment 1.3
No sympathy 1.2
Unexpressed resentment 1.15
Covert hostility 1.1
Anxiety 1.02
Fear 1.0
Sympathy 0.9
Grief 0.5
Victim 0.1
Hopeless 0.07
Apathy 0.05
Dying 0.01
Body Death 0.0

Getting better

Surviving

Succumbing

Getting worse

More significantly, each level of emotional operation carries a corresponding susceptibility to illness:

At 3.0, the individual is "resistant to infection and disease" and has "few psychosomatic ills" with an "interest in procreation."

Most people in society are operating at 2.5 and below—between apathy and boredom.

At 2.5, the individual is "occasionally ill, and susceptible to the usual diseases" with a "disinterest in procreation."

At 2.0, the individual has "severe sporadic illnesses," exhibiting a "disgust and revulsion to sex."

At 1.5, the individual has "depository illnesses (like arthritis)," has much anger, and "uses sex as punishment via rape."

At 1.1, the individual has "endocrine and neurological illnesses"

The message is clear. You cannot reverse aging if, by virtue of your emotional state, you are susceptible to illnesses that are deteriorating you. The solution: strive, by way of lifestyle, decisions and choice of responses to live higher up on the tone scale.

Note: I feel I must say this at this point. Don't let anyone's attempt to discredit the source or "kill the messenger" stop you from benefiting from the value in the message. See the full chart at https://www.agelessadept.com/resources

Why age reversal is, in fact, possible

"Aging is a belief that I simply don't agree with."

This is not about simply living longer. One of the "side effects" of clean cell living is that you can actually reverse aging and live longer in a state of youthfulness. I believe that reclaiming that state of youthfulness is, in fact, possible because....

Aging is a choice

In addition to the food we eat, there are ideas and beliefs we must transform in order to reverse aging.

Certain thoughts and ideas must be reconciled or rejected. To put in other terms, you must reconcile your mind with the essential truths and reject the lies.

The visible signs people associate with aging are simply conditions of the body. Conditions are effects. Effects arise from causes. Our causes are our actions. Our actions stem from choices. We make choices by agreement. Therefore age is an agreement. We age because we've agreed to it. (Read that again!)

Now, here's what I mean by "agreement." The only reason aging is inevitable is because we all agreed to it as one of a few limited choices. In other words, once we reach a certain age, we look around and ask ourselves, "What does it mean to be twenty, thirty, forty or fifty?" We become whatever we see as society's answer. We choose our new age-appropriate identity based on what others—typically family, friends, and others —say and show us to be the norm.

If, however, you created a new thought form of what thirty, and forty and fifty represent, you could achieve different effects. Challenging but doable.

Those causes and effects are under your control. Everything we believe about health and aging are thoughts planted from outside ourselves. The Seven Conversations help you see different choices. The Seven Conversations help you replace those thoughts with new ones and thus help you make new choices.

You choose to survive or succumb by your choices. Therefore, you must constantly choose youth. Sustain that choice, and you create immortality. It is possible to travel the "Backward Path" to agelessness.

People say that we each have a certain amount of "life energy" at birth that we use it up as we age; that once that energy goes, then so do we. They ask, "Can we really keep choosing youth indefinitely?"

My response is that long life and immortality are functions of belief. There is no reservoir of life energy you withdraw from, there's no tank to deplete. As long as you are alive, you have complete, total access to the full range of life energy required to support life. There is no such thing as being half-alive.

However, there *are* people who seem less full of life than others. There are those whose life energy seems to be decreasing as they age. Why is that?

The answer is quite simple. Let's think about children for a moment. It's more than their innocence, or their excitement with the world that set children apart. Children have a zest for life because the future is unknown. Do you remember how the days seemed interminably long when you were a child?

Days seemed longer and loomed in our minds as undefined, unknown things. You could lie in bed at two in the afternoon staring at the ceiling daydreaming because 3:00 pm held no requirements or limitations on you or on itself. Time seemed to stretch on forever because the present held no requirements. You had no concept of obligation, rent, taxes, appointments or disappointments (i.e., the "known" things that fill the minds of adults). For you, life was a big "unknown."

However, as you got older and were given more responsibilities, present moments like that 2:00pm siesta got interrupted more frequently. You spent less time being in those unknown moments, and more time anticipating and planning for your new, exciting set of known moments. Those present moments got shorter the more you focused on the future. Mentally, that's when your childhood ended. Youth ends when the experience of living in the infinity of today's real "now moments" gets replaced with anticipating the finite spans of more and more unreal "tomorrow moments."

The result: you spend less time in the present. From a mental perspective, youth and immortality exist in the present moment mind. I don't mean that figuratively or abstractly. Let me share how I knew I was getting younger, and how you will know too.

It was many years ago, and I had already spent years replenishing and releasing the physical elements my body needed to sustain youth. I had also spent years releasing thoughts, possessions, constraints on my time, obligations to employers, car payments, debts and created a lifestyle of freedom "off the grid."

One morning I woke, opened my eyes, and found myself staring at the ceiling. I had no job to go to. I had no bills to pay. I had no specific reason to rush out of bed that day. I was living my ideal life of minimal obligations and minimal possessions, and didn't have a plan of 'must dos' for that day. For a fleeting moment, I reconnected with a feeling I hadn't felt in years—it was vaguely familiar since I'd not experienced it since I was about seven years old. It lasted only a few seconds, but it was palpable, and I was excited beyond belief! It was at least a month before it happened again. And then it happened again a few weeks later.

Eventually, the feeling became more frequent and lasted longer. Today, I live it almost continuously. And on those days that I get caught up in the swirl of society, I can always return to that feeling at will with just a conscious thought. But it was on that day that I knew the Backward Path was real, and that I was returning to prior states of cognition, awareness and being that had once been beyond reach. Yes, my friend, every prior state of being still exists along the path you took to get here. This is true because....

Opposites are extremes of the same thing

Understanding this simple, yet profound concept, can change your world. Consider this diagram:

```
darkness<--------------------------------------> light
```

(Fig. 2)

These extremes are opposites, right? However, they are nothing more than opposite ends of the same "thing." Darkness is nothing more than the progressive reduction of light. You get to darkness by reducing the light. Similarly, take any set of opposites (black & white, up & down, rich & poor) and you can see that they are really two points on a line. That line is what I mean when I say the same "thing."

```
scarcity<----------------------------------------> abundance

acid     <----------------------------------------> alkaline

apathy <----------------------------------------> enthusiasm

low vibration<------------------------------------> high vibration
```

(Fig. 3)

Similarly, disease and health are two extremes of the same "thing." You get to disease by taking progressive steps away from health, and you get to health by taking steps away from disease.

This is profound. It means everything is a process, a trend. It means every state of being is part of a gradual progression. It means there exists a definable, observable path from one point to the next towards its opposite. I can change poor into rich by doing specific things that move me in the direction of richness. I can change down to up by moving in the direction of up.

Now, here's where it gets a little challenging for most people, yet the law holds true just the same: I can move from the conditions that are associated with "aging" towards the conditions associated with "youth" by doing certain things, by stopping and reversing the beliefs, thoughts, words, actions, habits and practices that have contributed to this point on a line called "aging." Yes, this means that everything is reversible, and it also means that while the increase in your collection of "years lived" might be inevitable, the conditions associated with that collection of years don't have to be. This is true because....

Aging is simply a bad habit

Now, let's take a closer look at that line. Imagine that your health at any single moment in time is represented by a single point along that line. Let's say this line has 26 points each represented by the letters of the alphabet. Your health journey, therefore, would look something like this:

A B C D E F G H I J K L M N O
--»»

Further, let's say that position "G" represents a few specific symptoms of aging (eg. gray hair)

As you go through life living your habitual lifestyle, certain accumulations and depletion occur, the flow gets blocked, and you begin deteriorating and progressing along this line—moving further and further to the right. Perhaps at age 30, you start experiencing some "A" symptoms, then a few months or years later, some "B" symptoms. By the time you start noticing full blown "G" symptoms (graying hair), you may already be at point J, K or L on the path.

In other words, starting many years ago, you got into the bad habit of aging, and now it is starting to manifest visibly!

Furthermore, this systemic deterioration will usually have numerous other manifestations beyond just your "G" symptoms. In other words, by the time you get to "G" and beyond, there could be many "invisible" conditions affecting your overall health.

For example, by the time you get to "G" and beyond, you may have accumulated heavy metals in your organs or blood. You may have accumulated worms and other parasites in your organs, blood or system. You may have the accumulated effects of an overly acidic system--a condition that causes free radical damage and ultimately devolves into cancer. You may be depleted in several critical nutrients, enzymes, vitamins and minerals. Or, you may have a depleted digestive, endocrine, nervous, lymph or other vital system. We could go on.

The point is that cure cannot simply be about addressing your "G" symptoms. Dyeing your hair doesn't reverse aging. It simply masks a symptom. The only way to reverse aging is to somehow get back to point "F" which is where you were, say at age thirty, just before your "G" symptoms started to appear, and then continue backwards to prior points. The objective of the Clean Cell practices is to halt this progression, and reverse the overall trend and the direction of your journey along this path. This is possible because...

All prior points are achievable

You are what you are at age forty-three because of what you were at age forty-two plus the effects of a year's worth of thoughts, words and actions. Again, age is an effect. The effect you refer to as forty-three years of age is the effect of age forty-two plus certain causes. Similarly it can be defined as "effect forty-four" minus certain effects. Does this make sense?

Every prior state/condition or point on a trend exists as an achievable state of being. This is true because of what we've already learned: that illness is simply a function of accumulation and depletion— something inside the body that shouldn't be there, and/or something that should be there that isn't.

Therefore, if you are on a point on the line closer to "illness" and if you find yourself moving to the right and feeling out of balance today because of something you ingested, you can return to yesterday's condition by allowing that thing to pass out. Similarly, if you feel out of balance today because of something that is depleted, you can return to yesterday's condition by replenishing that thing. You can do this because...

Everything is reversible

The fact that people *do* heal; that people's cancers can go into remission; that people *can* test positive for something today and test negative tomorrow; that people *can* cure incurable diseases, means that prior states of health are attainable.

Yes, it's like going back in time. If you arrived at point "I" by eating French fries every day, then to start reversing the trend, it is simply necessary to stop eating French fries, and to take some remedial action as well. There is no way around it. Your present condition is the direct result of actions you have taken —things done as well as things not done. Therefore, reversing these actions and non-actions is the only way to truly reverse your condition! Please read that statement again and embrace it. It holds the key to your success reversing aging the clean cell way.

By addressing the release of accumulation and the replenishment that true health requires, and allowing your body the time it needs to naturally heal itself, you will be strengthening your immune system, correcting imbalances, ridding yourself of parasites, reducing your body's level of toxicity, acidity, and as a result you will stop and reverse the body's deterioration.

I know this may seem like a tall order, but remember: the body is naturally coded to heal. All you have to do is support it naturally, and allow it the time and environment to do what it is already coded to do.

Now, this "cure" isn't for everybody. There are many   individuals   who   are   battling   serious, physiological and psychological addictions that present major challenges to implementing this solution, and this is not meant to trivialize their realities. That aside, our "magic dust," "overnight fix" society encourages people to opt for what they hope is a quick remedy. Again, this is a matter of personal choice. You are free to make any choice at all. Just remember, however, that every choice has consequences.

Now let's continue this line of thought. If sickness can be transmuted into health, then it stands to reason that age can be transmuted into youth. Why? Because, as we've already stated, the visible signs we associate with age are simply words we use to define a condition of the body. And just like any other condition we experience, it has certain causes.

Since we learned that any condition is a point on a trend, then youth and agelessness--as points on the path on the opposite side of age and demise--are states of the body and mind due to certain causes.

Agelessness—"yesterday's you"—like any bodily condition, is the predictable, achievable result of specific actions. Fortunately, these actions and their opposites are knowable. I call it clean cell living.

Let me add something important. In this universe, there is no such thing as something "staying the same." The universe, as well as everything in it, is either contracting or expanding. As a physical being, you are contracting or expanding, improving or deteriorating, surviving or succumbing. If you are succumbing at a fast rate, you must stop that rate of succumbing, then sustain survival, then advance to prospering. Then you can start to reverse the trend in order to reclaim youth.

The Age Reversal Rejuvenation Hypothesis

Summary: If opposites are simply extremes of the same thing varying by degree; and if the state of your health is a point on a line of one thing; and if every prior point is achievable; and if bodily conditions can and have been reversed by going backwards along that line; and if aging is nothing more than a bodily condition, as well... then aging, too is reversible!

What age reversal is and what it isn't

We each have ideas, observations and expectations about what 'aging' means. Common questions and concerns include:
- *Is all this medicine you're suggesting safe for me?*
- *What cream can I use to get rid of wrinkles?*
- *Are you sure this diet will really work for me?*
- *Where's the science?*

• *Isn't aging inevitable?*

ANSWER: This is not about medicine or drugs

Hippocrates said: "You can't cure cancer with a Happy Meal, silly!" or words to that effect.

This is not "medicine" in the way it is typically perceived in our society: *"an unnatural, chemical, off-the-shelf concoction taken to address a particular disease, which is then placed back on a shelf as the individual returns to the decadent lifestyle that originally caused the disease."*

The specific items recommended in this book are not drugs or chemicals created in a laboratory. They are all based on food. Real food. And in the same way you didn't ask for permission to eat the junk food you may be addicted to, you don't need anyone's permission to eat a fruit or vegetable.

As one author astutely noted, *"Illness is not caused by a deficiency in drugs, therefore, drugs cannot be the answer to health." No one says, "I just discovered I have a Prozac deficiency, so I need to take Prozac."* How on earth can putting foreign, unnatural, non-food chemicals in the body restore health? That's just patently absurd.

ANSWER: Creams? this is not about cosmetics

The glow of agelessness and beauty cannot come from the outside. Yes, you can moisturize the skin, use chemicals to color, correct and conceal blemishes and signs of aging, and topical applications of coconut oil and grapeseed oil and vitamin E can do wonders to hydrate, purify and cleanse the skin. However, age reversal is not a cosmetic thing. You cannot lather on youth. Youth is a function of the body's biological age. That biological age is a function of your internal biology, not pharmaceuticals. True youth is internal.

ANSWER: Diet? This is not a diet

Yes, half the clean cell concept revolves around food. However, this is not a "diet" in the same way that the word is perceived in our society: *"a bland departure from a fun and tasty 'normal' lifestyle that I must embark upon to lose weight or avoid my second heart attack."* No, this is, and should (and hopefully will become) your normal, tasty lifestyle! While we're on the topic, here's something to consider about the inherent contradiction and fatal flaw in all diets and why it is often difficult to adopt a new way of being.

When it comes to dieting, one of the reasons it is difficult for you to break free from your habits is that the vibrational level of who you are at any given moment is affected by the thoughts you think, and the thoughts you think are directly influenced by the food you eat. In other words, it is difficult to escape the nature of thoughts that your food creates in you!

Let me say it differently. On a daily basis, you will typically entertain ideas, perceive options, and see choices of a nature that harmonize with the level of thoughts in your mind. If the brain is polluted with steroids and antibiotics and drugs and preservatives, it limits the range of thoughts you have, as well as the people you attract, and the circumstances you create.

So the very thing that pollutes you--your current diet--from which you wish to be free, prevents you from seeing clearly or having the will power to escape it. That's why this is challenging. Not impossible.

You are, in fact, what you eat. You think at the level of your brain's vibration. Your brain vibrates at the level of its cells. Your cells vibrate at the level of the blood that nourishes it. The blood vibrates at the level of the food you eat. It's a cycle.

It's no coincidence that people who stop eating meat feel calmer, less aggressive, and less chaotic. They start thinking different thoughts, which attracts different people and situations, and thus presents them with different options and choices.

So the best solution of how to help people find their disciplined selves is first to help them redefine who they want to be, find their own motivation and desire to make the necessary changes, and then help them to think from a different reality, for their thoughts alone can start them vibrating at a different level and move them towards the right path. (That's one reason I devote these opening chapters to the belief system before the actual nuts and bolts.)

ANSWER: Science? Where's your Big Mac science?

If you're apprehensive about trying any of these items and practices, I encourage you to step back a bit and ask yourself a few questions:

Whom did you consult before you walked into a fast food restaurant to consume their "food?" What double-blind studies did you insist upon before you purchased the MSG-laced frozen dinner you fed to your family? What credentials did you request before you put your child on drugs for hyperactivity?

Someone put a happy meal in front of you, and without batting an eye, you ate it, and asked for seconds! Someone puts tofu in front of you, and now you need to see "the science!" (I know you're not like that, of course, I'm talking about people you know!)

Well, the fact is, there is lots of science, anecdotal evidence, and testimonials to support all of what I suggest to you in this book, but you'll find little of it here. We don't need no stinkin' science! This knowledge is intuitive. Natural. Elementary. Obvious. This is deductive reasoning. You'll realize you were born knowing this, and that you don't need no stinkin' science to validate, justify or prove any of it!

Furthermore, the flaw in that word "science"—as it is used in our society—is that it puts the power in the hands of others who are presumably (but often not) more qualified to find answers. In other words, since we average people in society are not "scientists," it becomes necessary for us to wait for the scientists to research, prove and validate all of our decisions.

However, once you realize that scientists are themselves flawed--with their own gender and cultural biases, religious and political leanings, world views, personality disorders, cognitive shortcomings, often linear (not holistic) ways of thinking, subject to corruption by greed, prestige and the interests and dictates of the state and/or the highest bidder, then you realize the actually fatal flaw of giving control of your health to "science" and scientists.

Throughout history, "science" and its supporting governmental and economic structures have and continue to allow: mercury in teeth fillings, chemotherapy to treat cancer, fluoride in drinking water, pesticides in food, vaccines that cause autism, MSG in food, and have intentionally inflicted syphilis (and other) diseases on unsuspecting individuals.

My point is what we commonly refer to as "science" is not the sole arbiter—and in many cases, is the exact opposite--of validity, efficacy and truth.

Inevitable? Consider Biological age vs. Calendar age

I know what you're thinking: *"Isn't aging inevitable?"* The answer is "yes and no." While evolution and change are surely evident and inevitable phenomena in the universe, the forms that this evolution and change take are not inevitable.

When it comes to what we associate with aging —gray hair, low libido memory loss, wrinkles, loss of energy, aches and pains, weight gain, weight loss, and so on—none is absolutely inevitable. Bone loss is not inevitable. Memory deterioration is not inevitable. Loss of vitality and cognition are not inevitable aspects of being on the planet for extended periods of time. Common? Yes, but they need not be inevitable. Accepted? Yes, but need not be part of your reality.

Let me clarify what I mean by the term age reversal. This is important, because if you don't understand what we're actually doing here, you might miss the reality and the benefit of it entirely.

Think about this. Among the people who pass away due to "natural causes," why do some people's natural causes take them at 70, while others hang around until 102? Why do you think that is? Call it good genes or fate, but all other things being equal, it's nothing more than the condition a particular body is in at a given calendar age.

"Biological age" is a *qualitative* determination of how young your body is regardless of your "calendar age" (number of actual years lived). You can have been on the planet for 50 years and have the biological age--with the libido, energy, functionality, glow and stamina—of someone in their twenties.

You see, we both may be 102, but our bodies deteriorated at different rates along different paths, and we ended up in different conditions. My body can do what a twenty-year-old's can. That means I have the age-appropriate functionality of a twenty-year-old.

Now, if I give you a tonic that washes away the deposits in your joints so you can move your fingers with the freedom and flexibility you had the year before, or even last month, then your hands have effectively gotten younger. It's not semantics, or a play on words. It's real, and what age reversal is all about-restoring the mobility, clarity, bodily function and flexibility associated with their younger years.

That's what we'll be doing: helping you clear away the "stuff" that has robbed you of that earlier clarity, mobility and ability, and offer instead the right stuff to create freedom, function and fun!

Reframe the challenge
In 2001, Takeru Kobayashi entered the Coney

Island hot dog speed eating contest. The record at the time was 25¼. However, in a single 12 minute competition--his first--Kobayashi blew through the record and ate 50 hot dogs to claim victory! Doubling a long-standing record your first time out is an amazing feat. Before Kobayashi, contestants asked themselves "How do I fit more hot dogs into my stomach?" Kobayashi, however, asked "How can I make one hot dog easier to eat?" He dissected the physical action of eating and optimized it for speed and efficiency. By reframing eating as a sport, asking a different question, and operating from a different paradigm, he changed what was possible and now others are eating 50 and 60 hot dogs!

Overlooking the fact that this is about a competition involving an item you won't ever be eating if you follow the Clean Cell practices, his story may inspire your own paradigm shift. Perhaps, while everyone else is asking *"How can I add more years or live longer through kryogenics, DNA manipulation or some other pharmaceutical-based technology?"* ask *"How can I keep my body clean inside and out so it doesn't age the same way others do?"* Perhaps you will, like Kobayashi, succeed in doubling life's record!

CHAPTER 4: Interlude ▲
Something to think about

What does health look like?

I'd like to challenge you to a little mental exercise. What do you think about when you think about healing a disease? In other words, what do health, healing and cure look like to you? If you're like many people, the images that come to mind include: orange bottles with white labels, multi-colored pills, white lab coats, masks, high-tech machines in sterile rooms, chemotherapy, intravenous drips and the hair loss it often causes, hypodermic needles, patent-infringement cases and thousands of dollars in cost.

Is this the way it has to be? Is Nature that flawed and imperfect? Is that the best our society can do as a solution? Or, is there another way?

Is there a way to heal and cure, reverse and rejuvenate an individual's body from deterioration and illness, without the use of harmful chemicals, radiation, invasive surgery, bodily dismemberment, mutilation, side effects and hair loss?

Following is a collage of the images most people call to mind when thinking of healing:

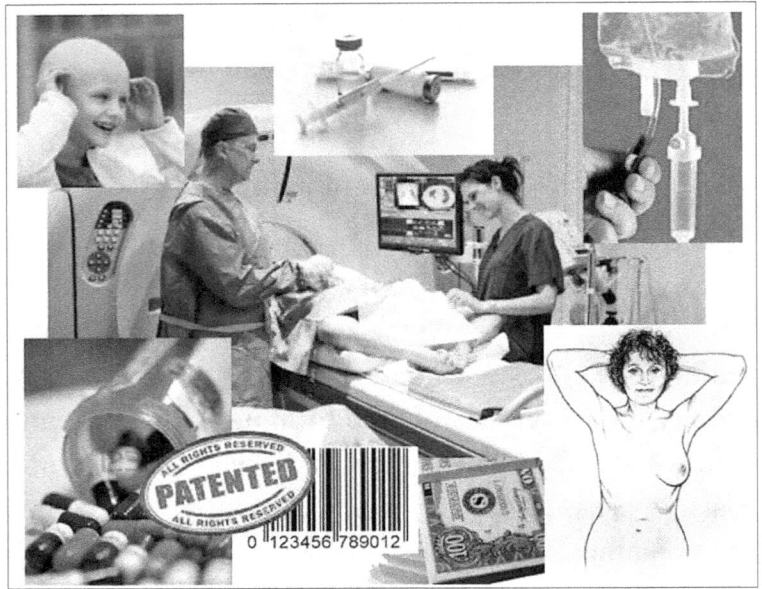

The old paradigm of healing
(Fig. 4.)

I suggest to you, however, that in the search for a better belief system, and in the quest to reverse aging, become fit to breed or simply live a healthy, long life using these practices, that you re-imagine what healing and cure—in reality—look like.

Perhaps healing and cure really look like this: Sunshine, clean air, clean water, direct contact with the earth and soil and access to real organic food without fear of patent infringement, all achieved for pennies. Here is that image:

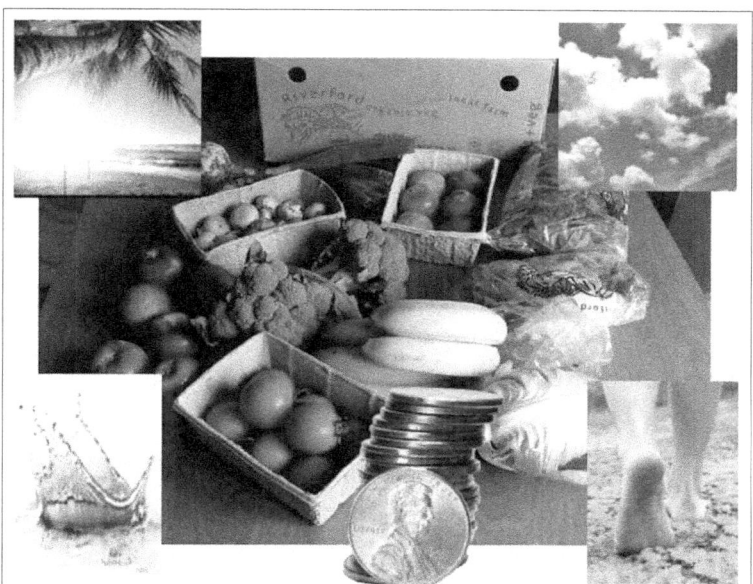

a new paradigm of healing. Something to think about.
(Fig 5.)

Art imitates life

A year after I published *The Man Who Lived Forever,* a great movie came along called "The Man from Earth" based on Jerome Bixby's book about a man who survives from Cro-Magnon times until the present. It has become a cult classic.

In the movie, one of the characters with a medical background, posits the possibility as well as what it would require for that sort of agelessness to occur:

Harry: "...it could happen. The pancreas turns over cells every twenty-four years, the stomach lining in three days, the entire body in seven years, but the process falters. Waste accumulates, [and] eventually proves fatal to function. Now, if a quirk in his immune system led to perfect detox, perfect renewal, then yeah, he could duck decay."

Edith: "That's a secret we'd all love to have!"

Well, I can tell you and Edith, from personal experience, that the secret is not a mystery. There are realities I've proven and results I've created for myself and others, for which I didn't need a medical degree, the validation of scientists, the approval of government, or reporting by the six-o'clock news:
• I've reduced 20-year old scar tissue with DMSO.
• I've cured my own tooth pain with clay and MMS.
• I've kept my stamina/ virility at college-age level
• I've cleansed my blood to get rid of slowly creeping black spots that were appearing on my face
• I've cured my own worsening colitis
• I've helped a pre-menopausal woman to regain bright red menses, a youthful glow, and the attention of men and women on the street!
• I've helped a friend regain mobility and eliminate years-long chronic pain with a 10-day water fast
• I've helped male friends regain their libidos
Yes, contained within the strategies of the Clean Cell Protocol is that "secret" we'd all like to have!

The Myth of Modern Medicine
or "Why they'll never find the cure for cancer"

The paradigm and belief system upon which modern medicine and its support system are based are polar opposites of the clean cell philosophy and are based on several illusions. *They* believe (a) Nature is flawed, (b) health is random, (c) you can and should eat anything that tastes good, (d) supermarkets are in the business of selling food, (e) pleasure and instant gratification are sustainable lifestyle modes, that (f) government agencies and pharmaceutical companies exist to help us and (g) the individual is unqualified to be his/her own authority--paving the way for institutions to prey upon public ignorance, fear and learned helplessness in the face of illness and cure.

Additionally, modern medicine employs a treatment paradigm that seeks ever to kill "the malevolent microbe." They treat symptoms rather than causes, cut and remove rather than cure and restore, and over-prescribe antibiotics and chemotherapy.

Society, meanwhile, subsists on three or more meals per day--plus all the snacks you can eat--made from genetically modified, poorly combined, canned, denatured, overcooked, nutritionally devoid fast food.

This is the direction medicine and society have been heading for generations--a path that leads to a host of familiar outcomes: Alzheimer's, rapid aging, impotence, overweight, low energy, high cholesterol, heart disease, cancer, etc. Here's what that looks like:

Effects	Food Paradigm	Treatment Paradigm	Belief System
• Alzheimer's • Cancer • Rapid aging • Imbalance • Low energy • Pain • High cholesterol • Impotence	• 3+ meals per day • Genetically modified • Fast food/TV Dinners • Canned • Preserved • Denatured • Overcooked • Poorly combined	• Treat symptoms • Cut and remove • Antibiotics • Chemotherapy • Pharmaceuticals • Patent-driven	• Nature is flawed • Health is random/luck • Freedom of choice • Supermarkets sell food • Instant gratification • "They want to help me" • Fear and powerlessness

While everybody's running to the left...

Are you running to the left? (Fig.6a)

Meanwhile, a few people are running in a different direction. *We* believe (a) Nature is perfect (and foolproof), (b) health is an effect (c) the body is coded to heal (d) health requires real food, (e) Nature has its own pace for healing, (f) corporate capitalism--not public well being--has been the prime directive, and (g) the empowered individual can be his/her own authority in personal health.

Our belief system's healing paradigm harnesses the preventive power of lifestyle changes; utilizes real food, sunlight, water, earth, air & time as the fundamental building blocks, and template for a system of proper nutritional support and removal of waste to create the necessary environment for health and longevity. Here's what *that* looks like as a comparable graphic:

Belief System	Food Paradigm	Treatment Paradigm	Effects
• Nature is perfect/foolproof • Health is an effect • Body is coded to heal • I eat only real food • Nature has its pace • No corporate capitalism • I am my own authority	• Real food • Organic, raw • Veganism • Mono meals • Caloric restriction	• Body healing • Cleanse & Purify • Nutritional healing • Prevention • Sunlight, water, earth, air & time • Enema, detox	• High energy • Vitality and libido • Freedom from illness • Youthful glow • Long life

...it takes courage and discipline to run to the right!

Or running to the right? (Fig. 6b)

Travelers on *this* path find high energy, vitality, relief from the effects of premature aging, and freedom from debilitating diseases.

One journey, fueled by advertising, consumerism, profits and patents is running conceptually "to the left." The other group, empowered by freedom and natural law is running "to the right." One group is essentially trying to find the north pole by heading south--seeking the rising sun by continually heading west. The outcomes are predictable.

This is why modern medicine will never find the cure they seek. Quite simply, they are on the wrong path. The cure already exists! It is known, practiced and already being experienced by thousands of people.

You can't cure cancer if you're not teaching people that cancer cells form in the *acidic* bodily environment and that the standard American diet of sugars, fried foods, dairy and meat creates, and that fruits and vegetables create an *alkaline* environment.

You can't cure cancer if you're not addressing the environmental causes--the magnetic fields, fluorescent lights, pollution, lead paint and pipes people are exposed to--and helping them to avoid them.

You can't cure cancer if you believe some miracle cure exists that can overcome cancer's causes and allow people to "enjoy" cancer-causing lifestyles while, at the same time, magically avoid cancer.

You can't "cure" cancer in the US if you outlaw any other treatment besides chemotherapy, forcing doctors to practice alternative therapies in other countries.

Neither health nor the cure for cancer exist down a road paved with fake food and chemicals, bathed in radiation and lasers, fueled by excess and greed, and motivated by corporate profits. No matter how many walkathons, telethons, gifts and grants are thrown at the ongoing research for "the cure," modern medicine will never find the cure for cancer because, it simply does not exist to be found on that road.

CHAPTER 5: Protocol ▲

pro-to-col – *n.* 1. a system of rules that explains the correct conduct and procedures to be followed in formal situations; 2. the plan for carrying out a scientific study or a patient's treatment regimen.

Understanding the basis of the protocol

We human beings are products of Nature. As such, our human coding is inextricably linked to the natural environment. We were designed to function optimally in an environment with specific ingredients in specific combinations. Air, sunlight, plant and animal life, minerals and ecosystems, were all designed to support each other and keep our innate healing codes activated. That's how it was for millions of years.

However, due to man's impact on the planet, everything from the earth's magnetic field, oxygen levels and air purity, ultra-violet rays, soil composition, to the planet's water supply have shifted into dissonance and disharmony. In other words:
- Our air is depleted and contaminated.
- Our soil is depleted and contaminated.
- We are not grounded by direct contact with the earth
- Our water is contaminated.
- We've been trained to avoid sunlight.
- Food is grown in depleted soil and unnatural chemicals
- What passes for food is not real.

As a result, there are certain levels of purity and balance that the earth is no longer able to create or sustain, and we are all feeling the effects.

We learn in school, for example, that the earth's atmosphere is 78% nitrogen, 21% oxygen and 1% inert gases. New evidence shows those weren't always the percentages. Our atmosphere was once closer to 50% oxygen. Certain parasites, which could not thrive in oxygen-rich environments—the environment of past eras—now thrive and multiply out of control. Think what effect that has on your body, the bloodstream, plants, and the existence of parasites in the system.

Such changes move us out of balance with the natural order, and suppress our body's healing codes. Therefore, anything you can do to return your body and its environment to the original pristine state— everything from putting plants in your home, using air purifiers, to eating organic food—all serve to reactivate your body's dormant code for healing.

The Prime Directive

pristine: adj. 1. In its original condition; unspoiled; remaining in a pure state; uncorrupted by civilization. 2. Remaining free from dirt or decay; clean. 3. Clean and fresh as if new; spotless.

Remember, Nature is foolproof, but we've lost that connection to Nature's foolproof perfection. The Clean Cell Protocol and lifestyle are simply compensating for the depletion in sunlight, water, earth and air, and our respect for time--and re-establishing that connection by replicating as much as possible a pristine, natural environment both internally and externally to bring things back now as they were then.

If things were now as they were then, you'd flood your body with oxygen by breathing clean fresh air. But, the way things are now, you need to oxygenate your water, take H202 or do oxygen therapy.

If things were now as they were back then, you'd wake up amid flowers in a natural setting. But the way things are now, you need aromatherapy to recreate and compensate for that condition.

If things were now as they were back then, you'd walk directly upon the earth and experience the benefit of the planet's magnetic field. But the way things are now, you use magnets to feel balanced and grounded.

If things were now as they were back then, you'd pick your food directly from the ground and ingest soil-borne organisms that would supply your intestinal tract with beneficial flora. But the way things are now, you need probiotics to keep your system balanced.

If things were now as they were back then, you'd walk to your destinations in the sun thereby creating a mild sweat that would detoxify your system. Now, you join a gym to run on a treadmill and sweat in a sauna.

If things were now as they were then, you wouldn't feel rushed to seek the overnight cure and the magic pill, and you'd trust and rely on Nature's pace to dictate the time it takes to cure illness.

Aromatherapy, hydrotherapy, homeopathy, acupuncture, fasting, magnetic therapy, oxygen therapy, even urine therapy work for many people and many conditions because they simply recreate conditions, vibrations and practices that once existed in Nature's perfection. If things were now as they were then, what we refer to as "therapies" would result as a natural part of your interaction with the world.

The "paradise paradigm" holds that the correct strategy for understanding the body and sustaining health, and the healing modalities that work best are those that replicate natural conditions that existed as it was back then (i.e., "paradise").

Therefore, the "prime directive" of the Clean Cell Protocol is to keep the body functioning as if living in such a pristine environment. Since there are fewer and fewer pristine environments for us to actually move to, we must compensate for the depletion in air, water, sun, earth and food, and replicate as much as possible, pristine, natural internal and external environments-our own paradise.

How to replicate paradise
(or create a reasonable facsimile thereof)

The cures or therapies in the Clean Cell Protocol are nothing more than variations on 5 themes:

1. sunlight
2. water
3. earth
4. air
5. time (SWEAT, for short)

All individual therapies, no matter how odd they seem, are variations on these themes. Let's explore:

How to replicate sunlight

The sun's ultraviolet rays are antiseptic and can kill bacteria, viruses, fungi, yeasts, molds, and mites in air and water, as well as on surfaces including our skin. It converts cholesterol in the skin to Vitamin D, and regulates bodily processes. Infrared rays improve neuralgia, neuritis, arthritis, and sinusitis. Sunlight regulates hormones and bodily processes, stimulates the pineal gland, and normalizes heart rate, blood pressure and respiration. It increases oxygen to the blood and thus improves muscular endurance.

Deficiency or insufficiency of natural sunlight and vitamin D has been associated with the following conditions: adrenal insufficiency, Alzheimer's, allergies, autoimmune disorders including multiple sclerosis and rheumatoid arthritis, cancers of the colon, breast, skin and prostate, depression, seasonal affective disorder (SAD), diabetes Type 1 & 2, gluten intolerance, heart disease, hypertension, Metabolic

Syndrome, infertility, sexual dysfunction, learning and behavior disorders, misaligned teeth and cavities, obesity, osteopenia, osteoporosis, osteomalacia (adult rickets), Parkinsons, PMS and psoriasis.

Don't let "conventional wisdom" scare you away from soaking in the sun! Soak for at least one hour each day; shorter duration for people with paler, melanin-poor skin.

There's no substitute for real, *direct* sunlight (i.e., there should be nothing between you and the sun except air; glass blocks the sun's infrared rays). However, here are variations to compensate:

Variations:
Infrared saunas, dry saunas, physical activity to encourage sweating, vitamin D supplementation.

How to replicate water

Simply drinking more and cleaner water can jumpstart your body's cure of itself and immediately increase your energy. Purified, fluoride-free, chlorine free, room temperature rain water would be best. Spring water is good. Reverse-osmosis, filtered water is good. Fill a container with half-gallon to one gallon each day and drink throughout the day.

Variations:

Drinking more water, hydrotherapy, purified water, ozonated water, oxygenated water.

How to replicate earth

In our modern world, and particularly in what Bob Marley called the "concrete jungle," it is possible for someone to be born, live and die without their feet ever touching the actual soil of the earth.

Think about it. They are born in a sanitized, concrete hospital. They are carried into and transported in a car that touches asphalt. They live their lives in high-rise apartments, and walk to school in shoes on cement sidewalks. They travel to work in steel trains. They live their entire lives--every waking and sleeping moment--separated from the earth hundreds of feet above the ground. And if, on that infrequent occasion they seek natural settings free of concrete or asphalt cover, they wear socks and slippers and sandals and shoes that separate them from the actual living earth. And, to take a few steps back in time, remember, they were even conceived and began the very instant of life in the womb of a woman who may never have touched the physical earth herself.

For many people, years can go by without them ever experiencing the grounding and rejuvenating effect of actually connecting to the earth.

What effect do you think that might have on the world view, thought processes, bodily functions, and even basic humanity of an individual, family or society who has never touched ground—people who are not, you might say, "grounded?"

In electrical terms, to "ground" an object means just that, to connect it to the earth. When an electrical appliance operates, for instance, it will build up an electrical charge. The earth naturally attracts excess electrical charge and dissipates it so that it does not accumulate and cause harm to the user. You ground something to keep it functioning properly and so it doesn't cause harm to itself or to others. I'll let you ponder, the significance of that statement as you consider that the radiation and unnatural magnetic fields of electrical appliances, power lines, cell phones/towers and x-ray scanners are all around us.

Variations:

Walking on the beach, touching soil, eating clay all keep you "grounded"; magnet therapy; clay baths.

How to replicate food

Just because something can be chewed and swallowed does not make it real food. I define real food as *"unmodified, raw, enzyme-rich nuts, seeds, fruits and vegetables eaten in as close to their natural state as possible."* Boiled carrots, or carrots from a can are not the same as raw carrots. If you can't put it in the ground and grow another one, then, generally speaking, it's not real food. *(Just because you're eating something out of a box with a picture of a carrot on the front doesn't mean you're getting the nutritional value of a carrot.)*

Variations:

Eating real food, organic produce, raw food, super foods, supplements, vitamins.

How to replicate air

You can go without water for a while, you can do without sunlight, you can even do without soil/food for many days. However, without air, you die in seconds. Therefore, since air is arguably the most important element, when looking to heal a specific condition, rejuvenate and grow younger, I suggest starting with air. As stated, there was a time when the oxygen content in air was as high as 50%. Now it's less than 20% and even lower in major cities. The more you can do to introduce oxygen into the system, the more optimally the body will function.

That's why one of the first things I suggest to my friends who seek my advice is to start taking daily supplementation with food grade hydrogen peroxide H_2O_2 actually increases oxygen uptake in the body.

Variations:

H2O2 (Hydrogen Peroxide), DMSO, Ozone therapy, MMS.

How to utilize time

Nature has its own pace for healing. The way to activate Nature's healing pace is to stop eating--to engage in an extended fast--to allow the body's healing code to take over and to heal itself. There is no way to replicate time.

Directive #2: Keep the body clean

As we learned, a clean cell never dies. Consequently, the overriding thought that should pervade your consciousness and intention as you live your life is *"How can I keep clean?"* Not "clean" in a fastidious, germophobic, neat-freak way—for if you visit my own home, you'll find I'm more a minimalist Oscar Madison than a Felix Unger —but clean in the sense of keeping the cells and tissues of the body free of bacteria, mold, parasites and toxins. I do this by being vigilant about what I put on my body, what I put in my body, what I put in my mind, and what environments I allow myself to dwell in. More later.

Directive #3: Replenish

96.5% of the body's weight is water. This includes Carbon Dioxide, DNA, RNA proteins, lipids and sugars composed primarily of Oxygen (65.0%), Carbon (18.5%), Hydrogen (10%) and Nitrogen (3%). The remainder is various salts comprised of Calcium (1.4%), Phosphorus (1.1%), Potassium (0.25%), Sulphur (0.25%), Sodium (0.15%), Chlorine (0.15%), Magnesium (0.05%), Iron (0.006%); Trace amounts of Chromium, Cobalt, Copper, Fluorine, Manganese, Molybdenum, Selenium, Tin, Iodine, Vanadium and Zinc. These must be replenished for the body to retain youth, elasticity, immunity, vitality, energy, regenerative capacity, and structure over time.

We lose these elements through ejaculation, menstrual flow, sweating, defecation, urination and even breathing.

Science does not know everything that is required for the body's function. There are compounds, solutions, molecules (i.e., combinations of individual elements), in specific amounts affected by interaction with others, under specific conditions, the purposes of which Nature has not divulged. Therefore, obtaining your nutrition for replenishment is best done by eating real foods and living as naturally possible so as to benefit from Nature's kept secrets.

Directive #4: Maintain alkalinity

Principle: the body functions best in alkalinity

Scientists use a measurement called the "pH scale" for measuring the acidity or alkalinity of various substances. (pH mean power of Hydrogen). The pH scale ranges from 0 to 14. Lower numbers indicate a more *acidic* concentration and higher numbers are more *alkaline*, with 7 (the pH of pure water) being the neutral midpoint. The ideal pH of the human body is not 7, but is actually 7.365 (above neutral/slightly alkaline). Once outside of this range (either too acidic, or even too alkaline), the body's metabolism goes out of balance (i.e., too much alkaline is not better!) As a result of consuming sugar, meat, dairy, fried foods, etc.—most of us are very acidic.

If the diet doesn't contain enough alkaline minerals to nullify the body's acidity, acids accumulate and the body is forced to "borrow" alkaline minerals — calcium, sodium, potassium and magnesium—from the organs and bones in order to neutralize the acid and remove it from the body. That's why people can drink cow's milk (acidic) all their lives "for calcium" and end up with osteoporosis. Remember, the body is coded to heal and is always invoking its natural intelligence to rebalance itself.

All this excess acid as well as the effort to rebalance strain the body. The result is acidosis, a syndrome that can cause cardiovascular damage, weight gain, obesity, diabetes, bladder failure, kidney stones, immune deficiency, free radical damage, hormonal imbalances, joint pain, aching muscles due to lactic acid buildup, low energy and chronic fatigue —everything we associate with aging.

Other symptoms include slow digestion and elimination, yeast/fungal overgrowth, low energy, low body temperature, infections, depression, anxiety, headaches, loose and painful teeth, inflamed and sensitive gums, stomach ulcers, cracks at the corners of the lips, excess stomach acid, gastritis, thin brittle nails, dull hair, dry skin, leg cramps and spasms.

One of the best ways to help rebalance the body to be more alkaline is to eat foods that are more alkaline-forming. This will help keep the body's pH level in a healthy 7.35-7.45 range. Choose a diet 70% alkaline and 30% acid, at least when you first start on the road to health. As you become more balanced, a more desirable ratio is 60% alkaline and 40% acid. But don't worry too much about ratios and proportions. Most people are so imbalanced toward the acidic side of the food scale, that simply eating a wide variety of real, raw food will do wonders to rebalance.

When we talk about acid and alkaline foods, we're not talking about the pH of the food itself, or the stomach acid or the pH of the stomach. We're talking about the end products the foods produce after digestion and assimilation. For example, a lemon is obviously acidic in its natural state, but when consumed, it results in alkaline end products forming in the body. Likewise, meat tests alkaline before digestion but leaves very acidic residue in the body.

When we digest a food, it is chemically oxidized (burned), to form water, carbon dioxide and a certain type of inorganic compound. It is the alkaline or acidic nature of this inorganic compound that determines whether the food is alkaline or acid-producing. If the compound contains more sodium, potassium or calcium, it is classed as an alkaline food. If it contains more sulphur, phosphate or chloride, it is classed as an acid food. Refer to the following charts as it may not be intuitively obvious which foods are acid-forming and which are alkaline-forming. As you move **up** the list, the foods get less acid forming, (i.e., more alkaline-forming) and thus beneficial to health and wellness. As you move **down** the list, the foods get more acid forming. The simple directive, therefore, is: always eat high up on the food scale. And remember, you don't need anyone's permission to do so.

THE ALKALINE TO ACID FOOD SCALE

(Alkaline/acid properties of a range of foods, healthy and not!)
The body's healing code requires pH range 7.35-7.45 (Ideal 7.365)

EXTREMELY ALKALINE-FORMING (pH 9.0 to 8.5)

9.0: Lemons, Watermelon,

8.5: agar agar, cantaloupe, cayenne (Capsicum), dried dates
& figs, Kelp, Karengo, Kudzu root, limes, mango, melons,
papaya, parsley, seedless grapes (sweet), watercress,
seaweeds, asparagus, endive, kiwifruit, fruit juices, grapes
(sweet), passion fruit, pears (sweet), pineapple, raisins,
umeboshi plum, vegetable juices

Better ⬆

MODERATELY ALKALINE-FORMING (pH 8.0 to 7.5)

8.0: apples (sweet), apricots, alfalfa sprouts, arrowroot,
flour, avocados, bananas (ripe), berries, carrots, celery,
currants, dates & figs (fresh), garlic, gooseberry, grapes
(less sweet), grapefruit, guavas, herbs (leafy green), lettuce
(leafy green), nectarine, peaches (sweet), pears (less sweet),
peas (fresh sweet), persimmon, pumpkin (sweet), sea salt
(vegetable), spinach

7.5: apples (sour), bamboo shoots, beans (fresh green),
beets, bell pepper, broccoli, cabbage, cauliflower, carob,
daikon, ginger (fresh), grapes (sour), kale, kohlrabi, lettuce
(pale green), oranges, parsnip, peaches (less sweet), peas
(less sweet), potatoes & skin, pumpkin (less sweet),
raspberry, sapote, strawberry, squash, sweet corn (fresh),
tamari, turnip, vinegar (apple cider)
(Fig 7a.)

SLIGHTLY ALKALINE-FORMING (pH neutral to 7.0)

7.0: almonds, artichokes (jerusalem), barley-malt (sweetener-bronner), brown rice syrup, Brussels sprouts, cherries, coconut (fresh), cucumbers, egg plant, honey (raw), leeks, miso, mushrooms, okra, olives ripe, onions, pickles , (home made), radish, sea salt, spices, taro, tomatoes (sweet), vinegar (sweet brown rice), water chestnut

amaranth, artichoke (globe), chestnuts (dry roasted), egg yolks (soft cooked), Essene bread, goat's milk and whey (raw) horseradish, mayonnaise (home made), millet, olive oil, quinoa, rhubarb, sesame seeds (whole), soy beans (dry), soy cheese, soy milk, sprouted grains, tempeh, tofu, tomatoes (less sweet), yeast (nutritional flakes)

Better ↑

NEUTRAL ALKALINE-FORMING

Butter (fresh, unsalted), cream (fresh, raw), cow's milk and whey (raw), margarine, oils (except olive), and yogurt (plain).

Also alkaline: Meditation, Prayer, Peace, Kindness & Love (Fig 7b.)

VERY LOW ACID-FORMING (Neutral to 7.0)

7.0: barley malt syrup, barley, bran, cashews, cereals (unrefined with honey-fruit-maple syrup), cornmeal, cranberries, fructose, honey (pasteurized), lentils, macadamias, maple syrup (unprocessed), milk (homogenized) and most processed dairy products, molasses (unsulphured organic), nutmeg, mustard, pistachios, popcorn & butter (plain), rice or wheat crackers (unrefined), rye (grain), rye bread (organic sprouted), seeds (pumpkin & sunflower), walnuts

blueberries, brazil nuts, butter (salted), cheeses (mild & crumbly), crackers (unrefined rye), dried beans (mung, adzuki, pinto, kidney, garbanzo), dry coconut, egg whites, goats milk (homogenized), olives (pickled), pecans, plums, prunes, spelt

Better

LOW ACID-FORMING (pH 6.5 to 6.0)
6.5: bananas (green), buckwheat, cheeses (sharp), corn & rice breads, egg whole (cooked hard), ketchup, mayonnaise, oats, pasta (whole grain), pastry (wholegrain & honey), peanuts, potatoes (with no skins), popcorn (with salt & butter), rice (basmati), rice (brown), soy sauce (commercial), tapioca, wheat bread (sprouted organic)

6.0: cream of wheat (unrefined), fish, fruit juices with sugar, maple syrup (processed), molasses (sulphured), pickles (commercial), breads (refined) of corn, oats, rice & rye, cereals (refined), corn flakes, shellfish, wheat germ, whole wheat foods, wine, yogurt (sweetened)

EXTREMELY ACIDIC-FORMING (pH 5.5 to 5.0)

5.5: beef, carbonated soft drinks & fizzy drinks, flour (white, wheat), drugs goat, lamb, pastries & cakes from white flour, pork, sugar (white), beer, brown sugar, chicken, deer, chocolate, coffee, custard with white sugar, jams, jellies, liquor, pasta (white), rabbit, semolina, table salt refined and iodized, tea black, turkey, wheat bread, white rice, white vinegar (processed).

5.0: Artificial sweeteners

Better

Other highly acid-forming products:
Artificial sweeteners like (NutraSweet, Spoonful, Sweet 'N Low, Equal or Aspartame), barley, beef, Brazil nuts, breads, brown sugar, carbonated soft drinks, cereals (refined), chocolate, cigarettes, cocoa, coffee, cottonseed oil, cream of wheat (unrefined), custard (with white sugar), drugs, especially the cola type. To neutralize a glass of cola with a pH of 2.5, it would take 32 glasses of alkaline water with a pH of 10; fish, flour (white, wheat), fried foods, fruit juices with sugar, hazelnuts, hops, ice cream, lamb, liquor, lobster, malt, maple syrup (processed), molasses (sulphured), pasta (white), pastries and cakes from white flour, pheasant, pickles (commercial), pork, poultry, processed cheese, pudding, seafood, soft drinks, soybean, and sugar (white), table salt (refined and iodized), tea (black), tobacco, walnuts, white bread, white vinegar (processed), whole wheat foods, wine, yeast BS yogurt (sweetened).

Also acidic: Overwork, Anger, Fear, Jealousy & Stress
(Fig 7d.)

Directive #5: Keep the flow going

The underlying secret to perfect health, long life, and agelessness is the concept of flow. We are sickened and aged either by something that is in the body that shouldn't be there (accumulation) or by something that *should* be in the body that isn't there (depletion). The solution is flow.

To stay healthy, make sure there is consistent outflow of matter to match the inflow, and that nothing remains stuck *inside* the body that should be *outside* the body. The number of daily bowel movements should at least equal the number of times you eat per day. Now, it's best if your body performs these bowel movements on its own without "help," but sometimes it may be necessary to help it along with enemas, colonics or salt water washes or by ingesting bulking agents like psyllium husk fiber until the body is rebalanced. Don't let the sun set on a blocked system. You'll notice an increase in vitality and virility as you start having more bowel movements each day.

*

Just as Carrel did in his experiment, we will use two strategies for creating flow and keeping the body's cells clean: (1) provide nutrients; (2) remove waste.

Advice for those new to these practices

As you research these practices and products, you may read comments and forum posts from people who have performed or purchased them, as well as those who oppose them. For every 100 persons who claim a therapy works for them, you'll find a few who say *"this is a load of crap, you people are delusional and will hurt yourselves."* Such critique can often be enough to dissuade someone new to natural therapies. No one wants to appear naive or gullible.

Consider this: It's highly unlikely that 100 people in various countries woke up one morning and said, *"You know what? I'm going to make up a story about how a therapy helped me so I can dupe people into using it so they can hurt themselves,"* and then expended the time and energy to write stories for no benefit or reward other than tricking others. What's more likely (and common) are people who got up one day, stumbled upon alternative therapies that challenged their belief systems and reacted by ridiculing and shaming those who practice them. (You might even have such folks in your own family!)

You can have anything you desire if you have courage and discipline. Here's where courage comes in. Don't let anyone to talk you out of doing something to control your health! Let's start with removing waste.

SECTION II

CHAPTER 6: Waste ▲

The following practices eliminate waste.

| For some immediate results | 1. Squatting |
| | 2. Coffee Enema |

The necessary cleanses	3. Parasite Cleanse
	4. Colon Cleanse/Colonics
	5. Gall Bladder Cleanse
	6. Kidney Cleanse
	7. Liver Cleanse

| Deep cleaning and miraculous healing | 8. Sauna Detox |
| | 9. Fasting |

What they'll never teach in med school!	10. Urine Therapy
	11. Blood Cleaning
	12. Oil Pulling

A Word About Cleansing

Anyone serious about living a clean cell lifestyle must perform some specific cleanses to purge, detoxify, repair, heal and rejuvenate specific organs or bodily systems. The cleansing sequence--parasites first, then bowels/colon, then gall bladder, then kidney, then liver--is critical since it will remove the most toxins in the most sensible way. For instance, it makes no sense to do any cleanse if parasites (tapeworms, pin worms, ring worms, etc.) are living, breeding, laying eggs, reproducing and depositing their own eliminations and secretions within the very organs and systems you are attempting to clean. If your bowels are not removing waste properly, then the toxins that will be released in cleanses of the kidneys and liver will overload your system. Therefore, by cleansing the colon first and the kidneys second, the only toxins left will be the liver's.

The following are brief explanations of the various cleanses that exist. Research them online for more details on their benefits and correct procedures.

1. SQUATTING

When evacuating in the sitting position required by western toilets, the anal canal is pinched by the puborectal muscle and restricts easy evacuation. The result: strain, and a host of bowel diseases (hemorrhoids, appendicitis, polyps, ulcerative colitis, irritable bowel syndrome, diverticular disease, colon cancer, prostate disorders and bladder incontinence).

(Fig. 9)

Sitting versus Squatting

Rear

RECTUM

RECTUM

Anal Canal

To maintain continence the puborectalis muscle "chokes" the rectum

Squatting relaxes the puborectalis muscle and straightens the rectum

The posture humans have evacuated in for millennia--the most natural, which babies instinctively adopt--for which the body was designed and that most of the world still uses, is shown below. For those not able to squat in that position, various products can be crafted or purchased to raise the legs as shown below.

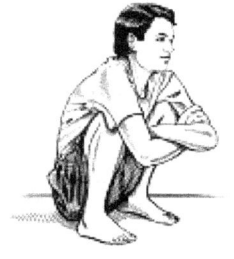

The relaxed, natural squatting posture

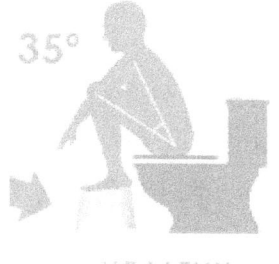

35°

HEALTHY

(Fig. 10)

You can't keep the cells of the body clean if you're allowing pounds of waste to remain un-evacuated. With this method, you'll find that your evacuations are easier (less strain) and more thorough and cleansing. This single change in habit can have a profound effect on your overall health.

2. COFEE ENEMA

Why you need it

Of all the "secret" practices in the Clean Cell arsenal, the coffee enema might be the single most impactful. Naturopaths recommend it. Charlotte Gerson uses it in her cancer-curing protocols and, prior to the advent of the drug age in modern medicine, it was even prescribed by doctors.

The liver is the body's second largest organ. Only the skin is larger. It is the largest glandular organ, and its size is in direct proportion to its importance. Without a healthy liver, a person cannot survive.

Among its functions, the liver secretes a substance called bile, which breaks down fats to make them more easily absorbed by the body. The liver also stores some of the body's vitamins and iron, converts sugar to usable sugar if the body's glucose level falls below normal, converts ammonia to urea, and destroys old red blood cells (if you've ever wondered why, under normal conditions, that no matter what you eat, your stool is typically that same brown color, it's because the destruction of old red blood cells produces waste that give it that color!)

However, detoxifying the blood of harmful substances is likely the liver's most well-known function. Whenever you ingest anything--from food to alcohol to drugs, and anything with chemicals, pesticides, etc.--the liver is taxed to filter it. You can see, therefore, how vital the liver is, and how, after years of filtering your blood of all manner of toxins in modern society and the standard western diet, it is likely to suffer the most and get clogged, weakened and abused. A coffee retention enema stimulates the liver to release these accumulations.

The history

Enemas are one of the oldest medical treatments known to man. The oldest known medical text, the Egyptian Ebers Papyrus (1,500 B.C.), records the use of enemas. Enemas were in use throughout the ancient world in Africa, Sumeria, Babylonia, India, Greece and China. Greek literature is filled with references to the therapeutic use of enemas. Egyptian pharaohs had a "guardian of the anus" a special doctor whose purpose (among others, I'm sure) was to administer the royal enema. Women in various countries in Africa use it on their children. American Indians, as well as preColombian South Americans crafted enema bags from animal bladders, latex and bones. For centuries, enemas were a standard home remedy in the United States as well, until their use died out.

Various sources, including: *The Royal Enema* by Dr. Ralph Moss

How and why it works

Enemas can be performed using water, herbs and other liquids. However, our protocol focuses on the coffee enema. During the enema, liquid coffee is introduced into the rectum to a place in the lower colon known as the sigmoid colon that contains a special circulatory system connected directly to the liver. The coffee only activates the liver, and does not circulate throughout the body.

The caffeine from the coffee is absorbed into this circulatory system and goes to the liver where it acts as a strong stimulant and detoxifier. It decongests the liver, causing it to dump its toxins. It also causes the liver to produce bile (which contains processed toxins from the liver) and stimulates the gall bladder to dump its contents that then flow directly to the small intestine for elimination.

The caffeine also stimulates the production of an enzyme used to form glutathione (an amino acid), which is one of the main substances that enable toxins to be eliminated via the bile into the small intestine. Therefore a coffee enema speeds up detoxification and minimizes the backlog of detoxified substances. You need a clean and well-functioning liver to keep your cells clean.

How to perform a coffee enema
This method uses an enema bucket. See *Master Shopping List*
[Resources] for this and other protocol essentials to keep on hand

What you will need
- 2 tablespoons finely ground organic coffee
- Unrefined coconut oil as a lubricant.
- 32 oz distilled or non-chlorinated filtered water
- Stainless steel, non-aluminum, non-coated pot
- An old towel, used only for doing enemas
- Enema bucket, bottle, bulb syringe or bag
- A timer

How to make the coffee.
- Put less than 1 quart water into pot and bring to boil
- Add 2 level tablespoons of coffee
- Let boil for 5 minutes
- Lower heat and simmer for 10 minutes
- Remove from heat, add balance of water to 32 oz
- Cool (or refrigerate ~10 min) to body temperature
- Strain the liquid by pouring it through a cotton cloth.

Always perform an enema *after* a bowel movement so the bowel is empty. Clean the bowels with a water-only enema immediately prior to the coffee enema. Your goal is two coffee enemas, not exceeding 2 cups each, held for 12 to 15 minutes. Don't worry if you can't hold for that long at first. Release as necessary, then try again. It gets easier.

How to administer the enema

Hang bucket about 2ft above floor; (You could also use a drugstore enema bottle; throw out the sodium phosphate—too harsh for regular use— and wash the bottle).

• Lubricate the tip of the syringe (end of tube) and the opening of the anus with coconut oil.

• Lie on right side, insert tip of syringe into anus

• Let the coffee drain into anus; If you use a small enema bottle, you'll have to squeeze, then unfurl, refill, and repeat (the bottle holds 4.5oz, so you'll need to do this approx 3-4 times)

• Lie on towel on the floor on your right side* with knees bent and close to chest; (i.e., fetal position)

• Set timer for 12 minutes. Do not change positions or do anything to cause the enema to enter deeper and further into the colon; this defeats the purpose of this type of enema.

• Hold inside for 12 minutes. Release in toilet.

Right side or left side?

As you research the coffee enema, you'll find sources advocating lying on your left side while others say right. Gerson himself and his daughter, Charlotte, say to lie on the right side. My naturopath said lie on the left, which made sense given the location of the sigmoid colon (the left). As a result, for years I've been doing left, and when I did my first enema, I could actually hear and feel the gallbladder squirt as my gallbladder emptied. These days, however, I advocate to lie on the right side.

Note: Both Gerson and my naturopath have been healing patients for years!

What to expect

Immediately upon releasing the enema, most people feel an instantaneous surge in energy, a feeling of clear-headedness and feel as if they've been instantly rejuvenated (and they have indeed). They simply can't believe that such a feeling is possible, and that a relatively simple procedure exists to achieve it. Even though the purpose of the enema is to stimulate liver detoxification, there is always usually a good amount of fecal material released during one's first enema. Many people are surprised at the amount of junk (the first few enemas can be quite foul smelling, too) that is inside them—believing that simply having a bowel movement a day was clearing the colon. (Wait until they actually do a deep colon cleanse!)

The coffee enema is just one aspect of the Gerson Therapy that has sent many types of cancer into remission.

A great overview is at
- www.hawaiinaturopathicretreat.com/procedures/gerson-therapy
- Visit Gerson.org for a video on the coffee enema.

3. PARASITE CLEANSE

Why you need it

You need it because whether you realize it or not, accept it or not, you likely have some form of parasite in your system. This may be true if you you've eaten meat, fish, sushi or even vegetables.

How it keeps the cells clean

A parasite cleanse removes these worms, their poop and eggs and other infestation from the colon, bloodstream and organs of the body.

How to perform one

There are several ways to do a parasite cleanse:

Specific Herbs

Taken over a period of time, wormwood, black walnut, quassia and olive leaf extract are known to eliminate worms and eggs. I've developed my own protocol combining an extended water fast, MMS (more later) that I've used to flush 16-inch worms from my system. There are products on the market (see Appendix) that provide combinations of these herbs.

Zapper

Hulda Clarke pioneered a unique technology for using electrical current to kill worms in the body.

See: www.parasitereport.com & parasiteblog.com

4. COLON CLEANSE

Why you need it

If your colon is obstructed, or if there is mucoid plaque (undigested, hardened fecal matter) lining the colon walls or trapped in the folds of the colon, you will be in a constant state of auto-intoxication, and will never fully absorb the nutrients in your food.

How it keeps the cells clean

A colon cleanse is a general term to describe hydrotherapy like colonics or a saltwater wash; bulking agents like psyllium husk, or combinations of various herbs that loosen the obstruction in the colon.

How to perform one

Colon Cleanse kits

Purchase kits that provide all the ingredients. See *Cleanse & Purify Thyself* by Richard Anderson.

Colonics

A naturopath or wholistic health center can administer a colonic--the introduction of water into the colon through the rectum for deep, thorough cleansing.

Fasting

Fasting allows the colon to rest, cleanse itself and return to its optimal state of functioning.

5. GALL BLADDER CLEANSE

Why you need it

The liver produces bile which helps with digestion in the intestines as well as elimination. Bile goes straight to the intestines or is stored in the gallbladder. Gallstones are solid particles that form from bile, cholesterol and substances in the gallbladder. You need this cleanse to keep those stones from forming.

How to perform one

From Ageless Remedies from Mother's Kitchen by Hanna Kroeger. Drink 8 ounces of apple juice at 8 am with 16 ounces to follow every two hours (10, 12, 2, 4, and 6). Be sure you are drinking natural juice, made without chemicals, eat nothing else that day. On the second day, repeat the apple juice schedule then at bedtime take 4 ounces of olive oil; you may flush it down with hot lemon juice.

How it keeps the cells clean

Despite what you've been led to believe, it is possible to remove gallstones naturally without resorting to removing the gallbladder. This and other cleanses allow your gall bladder to soften and empty its contents. A change in lifestyle and diet can keep it functioning normally.

6. KIDNEY CLEANSE

Why you need it

Every day, your two kidneys filter your blood of toxins, hormones, chemicals, and microorganisms, and also regulate fluid levels and hormones. A clean, well functioning set of kidneys plus an alkaline diet keep the blood clean and can reduce kidney stones.

How to perform one

A special tea (Hydrangea root, Gravel root, and Marshmallow root), along with Uva Ursi, Parsley, Ginger, Magnesium Oxide, Goldenrod tincture, Vitamin B-6, Black Cherry Concentrate are taken regularly for about 21 days.

How it keeps the cells clea

Despite what you may have been led to believe, it is possible to remove kidney stones naturally. This combination of herbs and vitamins functions to remove toxic accumulations from the nodules and fatty tissues of the kidneys and also promotes blood cleaning.

7. LIVER CLEANSE

Why you need it

The liver is considered the most vital organ and is the largest except for the skin. It receives blood directly from the digestive organs (the spleen, pancreas, and gall bladder), filters out waste and toxins, and converts them into substances carried safely out of the body. The liver is put under even more stress with alcohol, medication and all the other "non-food items" many people eat.

How it keeps the cells clean

The liver cleanse rejuvenates the liver and the gall bladder as well. We cleansed parasites, colon, gall bladder and kidney first so that the pathways of blood to the liver are now clean and toxins from those organs do not impede or overwork the liver's functioning.

How to perform it

Ingredients

- Apple juice or (optional) malic acid supplements
- 4 tablespoons of Epsom salts
- 1/2 cup of virgin olive oil
- 1 big grapefruit, or 3 lemons

Preparation

DAYS 1-5: For 5 days before your liver flush, eat as many apples, or drink as much apple juice as you can. Take malic acid supplements as an alternative. During the last 2 days, drink 8 oz apple juice every 2-3 hours.

<u>The day of the cleanse</u>

DAY 6: Eat a light, no-fat breakfast. This enables the bile in your liver to accumulate, putting pressure in your liver which will eliminate more stones.

2:00 PM: mix 4 tblspns of Epsom Salts in 3 cups of water in a jar. Do NOT drink or consume any foods after 2 PM. This is extremely important! The liquid may be refrigerated for drinking later.

6:00 PM: drink 3/4 cup of this mixture. You may add 1/8 tablespoons of powdered Vitamin C for taste.

8:00 PM: drink another 3/4 cup of the mixture. Get all your errands done now as you shouldn't do anything after drinking the 10pm preparation.

9:45 PM: pour 1/2 cup of virgin olive oil into a jar. Squeeze the entire grapefruit into the mix, removing the pulp. You should have 1/2 to 3/4 cups of this grapefruit juice/virgin olive oil preparation. Close the jar, and shake hard until it is all liquid.

10:00 PM: drink this mixture--through a straw if easier--all within about 5 minutes.

Lie down in bed *immediately*. Don't do any work, Don't brush your teeth. Don't clean up. Lay *immediately* on your right side, with your right knee up towards your chin for no less than 20 minutes. Stay very still and try to sleep.

The next morning

DAY 7: when you wake up, drink 3rd dose of your 3/4 cup Epsom salts. You may go back to sleep after.

+2 HOURS: drink the last dose of Epsom salts.

+2 HOURS: you may resume eating, but do not eat solid fruits just yet. Start with liquids.

What to expect

That same morning, you might experience diarrhea (caused by the Epsom salts). You may see a few (or hundreds of) gallstones in the stool. Green, floating, round pebble-like objects are gallstones.

Many people will *not* see gallstones in their first liver flush. Wait a week before your next liver flush. Some people may not see gallstones until their third or fourth attempt. Remember and respect Nature's pace.

See colonzone.org for more

8. SAUNA DETOX

Why you need it

Drugs and chemical poisons, the preservatives in food, atmospheric poisons, including pain pills, tranquilizers and diet pills, codeine, aspirin, Novocain, etc., and recreational drugs like marijuana, often remain in our bodies lodging in the fatty tissues for years. Even years after we've been exposed to or stopped taking these substances, we are still prone to experiencing their effects.

How it keeps the cells clean

Done correctly, a sauna detox--I call it a "hot rinse"-- can take you back in time to a state of clean cells! It uses exercise, vitamins, nutrition and time in a dry sauna to dislodge drug residues and other toxins from the fatty tissues so these substances can be eliminated from the body. Each session (exercise plus sauna) lasts approximately 1 to 1.5 hours.

Preparing your body

Make sure you are well hydrated. Stop eating 2 hours prior to the actual sauna session.

Your skin should be clean and free of any chemicals, soaps, oils or creams.

Make sure you are taking 2 or more tablespoons of fresh, organic, cold-pressed oil daily as well as fatty foods (olive oil and avocados are good). As mentioned, the toxins and drug residues seek out fats and lipids to attach themselves (that's why the brain, with its 70% lipid content, is a favorite target of drugs and chemicals). By increasing the available fat for these toxins to adhere to (oils and avocado), and then by eliminating the fat during the sauna, it makes it easier to eliminate toxins from the body. (If your blood cholesterol is less than 170, the sauna detox is not recommended, as you may not have sufficient lipids to protect the brain from outgoing toxins.)

Choosing a sauna

Steam saunas are not recommended because of the risk of fungal infections, and the burning effect of the steam, which tends to reduce the length of time people feel comfortable.

You can use your own sauna, one at your doctor's office, or at a public gym.

The recommended type of sauna is called a "far infrared" sauna as it encourages sweating at lower temperatures. This may not be practical because these saunas can range from $3,000 to $5,000 for the in-home versions. I use a stone-heated, dry sauna at my local gym.

What you'll need
- 2 to 3 large towels
- 2 to 3 hand towels
- flip flops/rubber sandals
- glass or polycarbonate bottle for hydration drink.

Plastic bottles leach toxins especially when heated.

Preparing the sauna

Prepare the sauna and preheat to between 120 and 160 degrees F. Higher is not better! Sweating is the important goal here, and you can sweat comfortably and quite profusely at that temperature (140 is ideal) without harming yourself.

If you use a public sauna, be aware of the risk of fungal infections. Do not touch the wood or floors (use towels and slippers at all times), and, if possible, do not use the sauna while others are present so as not to breathe in other people's toxic discharges.

Preparing your hydration drink
- 1 liter clean reverse osmosis or distilled water
- ½ teaspoon Ascorbate powder
- 2 capfuls of E-lyte electrolyte concentrate
- 1 scoop Red Alert by Doctors for Nutrition

Vitamin C helps the body eliminate toxins. Too much may cause cramping and diarrhea. The hydration drink is a very important part of the hot rinse sauna program.

Instructions

1. Take 100mg of pure niacin. Not niacinimide. Not "flush free" niacin, or time-released niacin.

2. At the same time, take:
two (2) Potassium citrate capsules (99mg each)

AND CHOOSE ONE OF THE FOLLOWING:

▶ three (3) Magnesium citrate caps (100mg) if you tend to have constipation, **or**
▶ three (3) Optimag 125 caps (125mg each) if you tend to loose stools.

3. Begin a 30-minute aerobic session (running on a treadmill, step machine, exercise cycle). The exercise is not for sweating. It is to encourage the circulation of blood, the dilation of blood vessels and to increase the amount of toxins loosened in the body. The exercise also allows the niacin and electrolytes time to enter your bloodstream. If you start to feel a tingle or a flush or heat, this is a normal reaction to the niacin.

4. After 30 minutes, stop the exercise and proceed immediately to the sauna. Grab your hydration drink, flip flops, towels and head straight inside as quickly as you can. Remove clothes. Sit on the towels (do not let your body touch the wood). Get comfortable and start

sipping your drink as you sweat. You should be drinking about one liter per 1/2 hour in the sauna.

If you're new to the sauna experience, start with 10-20 minutes and work your way up to 60 minutes over the next few saunas over the next several weeks.

Warnings

Everyone comes to the Clean Cell lifestyle at different stages of health and strength. Since there are real dangers involved if done too soon or incorrectly, I want to make sure everyone is well served by heeding these warnings. They are not meant to scare you, but simply to take into account everyone's unique strengths and weaknesses.

Because of the strenuous activity and high heat, do not attempt the hot rinse too early in your transition to clean cell living. Saunas mobilize toxins and sweating depletes minerals. Be sure your vitamin and mineral excesses and deficiencies are normalized first.

Liver, kidney and lymph systems should be functioning normally, and any colon issues and constipation should be resolved. These organs and systems are called upon to aid detox during the sauna.

NOTE: Even though you are becoming your own authority, if you are currently under the care of a health care provider, please consult that individual for advice as to whether your current condition and/or any medication you are taking may make you unsuited for vigorous exercise and high heat.

Leave the sauna immediately if you experience nausea, fainting or dizziness, swelling of hands or feet, cessation of sweating, blood pressure spike or drop, or mental confusion. Any of these may be signs of dehydration. If you experience muscle cramps, it means your electrolytes are insufficient.

Do not attempt to do this more than once a day. This is not meant to be an intense cleansing but an aid to health. There are clinics that offer this therapy for intense cleansing under supervised conditions.

For full and complete instructions, and warnings if any of the following apply to you (high blood pressure, past use of LSD or other psychedelic drugs, Multiple Sclerosis, breathing condition, prostheses, silicone implants or nerve damage), visit:. www.waltgoodridge.com/resources

How I do it

I go to the local gym to use their dry sauna since purchasing my own in-home sauna is not practical. I use running on the treadmill as my exercise. The sauna is heated by rocks, so I'll sometimes sprinkle a few drops of tea tree oil on the rocks in order to have therapeutic fumes to inhale. I typically use fresh, natural coconut water as the base for my hydration drink along with chlorophyll and lemons. I do the hot rinse perhaps once a month, or more frequently if notice any bumps on my skin that may indicate toxins in the system, and I remain in the sauna for half hour.

What to Expect

There may be different smells and sweat of different color that come to the surface during a sauna detox. You may smell chlorine (from water and previous swimming pool use), ammonia, as it leaves your body. Other people notice tastes and smells of food, chemicals and other substances they haven't actually ingested for years. One woman tells a story of seeing blue sweat coming to the surface and staining the towels blue. For years, she had worked in a paint factory and there was actually paint lodged deep in her tissues that was finally being released! Yes, a sauna detox can take you back in time!

9. FASTING

What it is

A fast is the act of consciously and intentionally refraining from eating solid food—drinking water only —for an extended number of days.

How it keeps the cells clean

The process of digestion we request of our bodies typically three or more times a day, is a very exhausting process. Fasting allows the body time to stop, rest, shift into repair and rejuvenation mode, during which it can accomplish some amazing things. Fasting is perhaps one of the most healthful practices for your body and overall health.

Fasting is Nature's first cure. It is consistent with our first principle that Nature is foolproof and designed so that even the least among us can access its power. Animals fast when ill. Humans, too, are often aware of a decrease in appetite when sick, and only need to listen to their bodies and refrain from eating in order to access Nature's foolproof healing power.

The process by which Nature heals during a fast is called autolysis (self-digestion, the destruction of a cell through the action of its own enzymes.)

The fasting body uses all its reserves of nutrients and fat, but also scar tissue, growths and obstructions, dead, dying and diseased cells, unwanted fatty tissue, trans-fatty acids, hardened coating of mucus on the intestinal wall, toxic waste matter in the lymphatic system and bloodstream, toxins in the spleen, liver and kidney, mucus from the lungs and sinuses, embedded toxins in the cellular fibers and deeper organ tissues, deposits in the capillaries responsible for nourishing brain cells and excess cholesterol...and even tumors!

[Yes,] *a remarkable phenomenon associated with fasting is seen in the many instances in which tumors, even tumors of considerable size, are autolyzed and completely disappear during a fast. Undoubtedly the nutritive materials of which the tumor is composed are utilized with which to nourish essential tissue, while the non-usable portions are cast out. In the process, the body is healed to an even greater degree.*

How fasting rejuvenates

Fasting is like "rebooting" your system! Beyond the amazing healing, there is also rejuvenation that is almost magical. Here are excerpts from the Rejuvenescence chapter of *Fast & Grow Young*, by Dr. Herbert Shelton who supervised the fasting of more than 40,000 people over a period of fifty years:

*

📖 Drs. Carlson and Kunde, of the department of Physiology of the University of Chicago, showed that a fast of two weeks temporarily restores the tissues of a man of forty to the physiological condition of the tissues of a youth of seventeen.

*

📖 By repeating the rejuvenating fasts at appropriate intervals, the individual can keep himself younger, year after year, much younger physiologically, than he would otherwise be, and, in short, stave off old age.

*

📖 E. Schultz, experimenting with fasting hydra, produced positive proof of the rejuvenating effects of fasting, the animals reverting to an embryonic state. Intensive nourishment results in much poisoning in infusoria and a short fast is needed to restore them to youth. A reduction of surfeit (an excessive amount of something; in this case, food) is essential to the most vigorous manifestations of vitality. In higher animals "brief hunger has a beneficial effect."

*

📖 Professor Child tells us [in] *Senescence and Rejuvenescence* (senescence is the condition or process of deterioration with age), that with abundant food some species may pass through their whole life history in three or four weeks, but when growth is prevented through loss of food, they may continue active and young for at least three years. "Partial starvation inhibits senescence. The starveling is brought back from an advanced age to the beginning of postembryonic life; it is almost re-born."

*

📖 It hardly need be said that in the larger and more complex forms of life the possibilities of rejuvenescence are more narrowly limited than among the lower forms such as the planaria (flatworm). Nevertheless, according to Prof. Child, in the organic world, generally, rejuvenscence is as fundamental and important a process as senescence.

*

📖 Experiments have shown that calves, when forced to fast, continue to grow. Although losing weight and becoming gaunt, they continue to increase in size, drawing upon their reserves and expendables for the nutrient materials and vitamins necessary to sustain growth in those portions of its organism that are growing at that stage of its existence.

*

📖 Excess is fatal to healthy action. A reduction of surfeit is essential to the most vigorous manifestations of vitality. Weismann's observations and the results of tissue-culture in the laboratory reveal that there are no limits to vitality. Autogenerated toxins and poisoning from gastro-intestinal putrefaction and fermentation are the chief limiting influences upon life. Surfeit produces and fasting eliminates these. A removal of toxins and surfeit permits tissue regeneration.

*

📖　Prof. Huxley, of England, son of the older Prof. Huxley, took some young planaria, or earthworms, and performed a very interesting and instructive experiment with them. He fed a whole family of these as they ordinarily eat. He isolated one of them and fed it in the same manner, but forced it to undergo at regular intervals, short periods of fasting. It was alternately fasted and fed. The isolated worm was still alive after nineteen generations while his brothers had been born, lived their regular life cycles and passed away. The only difference in the mode of life and the diet of this worm and that of his brother worms was his periodic fasts.

*

📖　An experimenter at the University of Chicago procured some insects of a kind, the normal life [span] of which is only twenty-four hours. He isolated them and placed them where they could not procure food. Instead of starving to death immediately or dying at the end of their normal twenty-four hours' life span, they lived for fifteen days. Fasting enabled them to live for fifteen generations.

*

📖　Now, these results obtained with worms and insects only forcefully remind us again that we cannot safely argue from one species to another. Man cannot live for fifteen generations by fasting nor for nineteen generations by periodic short fasts. Nor can he become a minute man by fasting and then, when fed, grow into a new and youthful man as was the case with worms.

*

     But there is a renewal of man's body to a certain extent. His body does become smaller. He does get rid of his surplus tissues, surplus food, accumulated toxins and "diseased" tissues, etc.

*

     A great change in cell life and structure takes place during a fast and it is well to continue the fast until this change is complete and nothing but healthy tissue remains. In this way a new body emerges from the process. It is thin, but ready to be re-built upon normal lines. After such an overhauling process, when the body has been largely torn down and thrown away, when the accumulated waste and debris of a life-time have been refined or cast out and, after the chemical readjustment, occasioned by the fast, has occurred, the body that is properly cared for is built anew and its youth renewed.

*

     Experiments upon human beings and dogs, performed at the Hull Biological Laboratory of the University of Chicago, and reported to the Journal of Metabolic Research, showed that a fast of thirty to forty days produces a permanent increase of five to six per cent in the metabolic rate. Note: A decrease in the metabolic rate is one of the phenomena of old age. Fasting, by increasing the metabolic rate produces, as one of its effects, rejuvenation. (emphasis mine)

*

📖 With toxin deposits cleared up; the body purified; the blood rejuvenated; organs renewed; senses improved; digestion and assimilation enhanced; the cells and tissues returned to a more youthful condition; infiltrations, effusions, and growths absorbed; dead and dying tissues removed and new tissues in their places; body chemistry normalized; the body is in very much the same condition as the mattress that has been to the factory for renovation and making over. After the fast has cleared away the accumulations and the devitalized cells, stronger, more vital and healthy tissue is built to take the place of that which was cast away. Regeneration of the body is brought about through the daily renewal of its cells and tissues and fasting hastens this renewal.

*

📖 On May 18th, 1933, one of the physicians attending Gandhi; during his fast at that time, reported that on that day, the tenth day of his fast, "despite his 64 years, from a physiological point of view, the Indian leader was as healthy as a man of forty."

Fasting is Nature's ultimate cure. Many animals—including household pets—refuse to eat when they are ill. The body diverts the energy it would normally use for digestion and assimilation, to the processes of healing and rejuvenation. It's been said there is as much of a 30% increase in the energy available for healing as a result of a fast. Societies have long advocated fasting for many ills. Read more in *Fast & Grow Young* available at www.fastandgrowyoung.com

Next, to understand the body's sequence of healing, let's take a look at exactly what happens during the stages of fasting.

The Stages of Fasting

Sources: *Orthopathy, Teaching New Science of Health & Natural Healing* by Shelton/Clements and *How & When to be Your Own Doctor.*

<u>Stage 1 (Day 1-2)</u>

On the first day of fasting, the blood sugar level drops below 70mg/dl (milligrams/deciliter). To restore the blood to the normal glucose level, liver glycogen is converted to glucose and released into the blood. This reserve is enough for a half day. The body then reduces the basal metabolic rate (BMR). The rate of internal chemical activity in resting tissue is lowered to conserve energy. The heart slows and blood pressure is reduced. Glycogen is pulled from the muscle causing some weakness. The first wave of cleansing is usually the worst. Headaches, dizziness, nausea, bad breath, glazed eyes and a heavily coated tongue are signs of the first stage of cleansing. Hunger can be the most intense in this period, but passes within a few days.

Stage 2 (Day 3 to 7)

Fats, composed of transformed fatty acids, are broken down to release glycerol from the glyceride molecules and are converted to glucose. The skin may become oily as rancid oils are purged from the body. People with problem-free skin may have a few days of pimples or even a boil. A pallid complexion is also a sign of waste in the blood. Ketones are formed by the incomplete oxidation of fats. It is suspected that the ketones in the blood suppress the appetite by affecting the food-satiety center in the hypothalamus called the appestat. You may feel hungry for the first few days of the fast. The desire to eat will disappear. Lack of hunger may last 40-60 days.

The body starts embracing the fast and the digestive system is able to take a much-needed rest, focusing all of its energies on cleansing organs and the lungs are in the process of being repaired. Periodically, the lymphatic system expels mucoid matter through the nose or throat. The volume excreted of this yellow-colored mucus can be shocking. The sinuses go through periods of being clogged, then will totally clear. The breath is still foul and the tongue coated with bad-tasting, dryish mucus, and urine may be concentrated and foul. The reason for this is "acidosis." During acidosis the body vigorously throws off acid waste products. Most people starting a fast begin with an overly acid blood pH from the typical western diet. Switching over to burning fat for fuel triggers the release of more acidic substances. Acidosis is usually accompanied by fatigue, blurred vision, and some dizziness. Within the intestine, the colon is being repaired and impacted feces on the intestinal wall start to loosen and are autolyzed.

Stage 3 (Day 8 to 15)

Many fasters feel more comfortable by the end of the first 7 to 10 days, when they enter the normalization phase. Here the acidic blood chemistry is gradually corrected. This sets the stage for serious healing of body tissues and organs. (usually it takes about ten days to two weeks of water fasting to seriously begin healing). Normalization may take one or two more weeks depending on how badly the body was imbalanced. As blood chemistry steadily approaches perfection, the faster usually feels an increasing sense of well-being, broken by short spells of discomfort (healing crises or retracings).

On this latter part of an extended fast, you can experience enhanced energy, clear-mindedness and feel better than you have felt since childhood, On the downside, old injuries may become irritated and painful. This is a result of the body's increased ability to heal during fasting. If you had broken your arm 10 years before, there is scar tissue around the break. At the time of the break, the body's ability to heal was directly related to lifestyle. If you lived on a junk food diet, the body's natural ability to heal was diminished.

During fasting, the body's healing process is at optimum efficiency. At about day 10, we enter the "Accelerated Healing" stage. As the body scours for dead or damaged tissue, the lymphocytes enter the older-damaged tissue secreting substances to dissolve the damaged cells. These substances irritate the nerves in the surrounding region and cause a reoccurrence of aches from previously injured areas that may have disappeared years earlier. The pain lasts as long as the body is completing the healing process. The muscles may become tight and sore due to toxin irritation. The legs can be the worst affected as toxins accumulate in the legs. Cankers are common in this stage due to the excessive bacteria in the mouth.

Stage 4 (Day 16 to 30)

The body is completely adapted to the fasting process. This is a miraculous time when tumors are metabolized as food for the body, when arthritic deposits dissolve, when scar tissues tend to disappear, when damaged organs regain lost function (if they can).

There is more energy and clarity of mind. Cleansing periods can be short with many days of feeling good in between. There are days when the tongue is pink and the breath is fresh. The healing work of the organs is being completed. After the detoxification mechanisms have removed the causative agent or renders it harmless; the body works at maximum capacity in tissue proliferation to replace damaged tissue. While a short fast will reduce symptoms, a longer fast can completely heal. Homeostatic balance is at optimum levels. The lymphatic system is clean except for a rare discharge of mucus through the nose or throat. After day 20, the mind is affected with heightened clarity and emotional balance. Memory and concentration improve.

Stage 5 (Day 30 and beyond)

The breath, which during all or most of the fast has been offensive, becomes sweet and clean. The tongue becomes clean. The thick coating which remained on it throughout most of the fast vanishes. The body temperature, which may have been sub-normal or above normal, returns to exactly normal, where it remains. The pulse becomes normal in time and rhythm. The skin reactions and other reactions become normal. The bad taste in the mouth ceases. Salivary secretion becomes normal. The eyes become bright and eye sight improves. The excreta loses its odor. The urine becomes light.

The primary indication that the fast is to be broken is the return of hunger; all the other indications are secondary. Often one or more of these secondary signs are absent when hunger returns, but one should not refrain from breaking the fast when there is an unmistakable demand for food, merely because the tongue, for example, is not clean. Inasmuch as all the signs do not invariably appear in each case, do not hesitate to break the fast when hunger returns.

Important caveat

Please note that not everyone experiences the full range and intensity of all the healing crises mentioned. Shelton was often dealing with individuals who came to him suffering from illnesses that made them very toxic. Your mileage may vary!

IMPORTANT: Do not overlook the significance of what you've just read. It is absolutely amazing that repair, reversal, rejuvenation and regeneration even after years and years of damage, bad habits and deterioration can be accomplished in mere days!!

The reason Shelton and others can create a "stages of fasting" guide that predicts with almost pinpoint accuracy what will happen to you during your fast, is that after guiding over 4,000 people, he realized the process is the same! Even a body damaged by years of abuse and neglect still retains its healing code.

If there were not this consistent, reliable, predictable thread of order in the universe, things would fall apart. If everyone's built-in code didn't function in the same way, Nature simply couldn't survive. A seed that fell into the soil, wouldn't know what to do! Birds that got cold in the winter wouldn't know where to go! Nature is, indeed, foolproof, and perfect! You are in good hands!

Juice Fasting

A juice fast is a good initial alternative to a pure water only fast. During a juice fast, the digestive system is not completely shut down as it is in a water fast, and thus the healing process is not as intense or quick. Dr. Isabelle A. Moser estimates that fasting on raw juices and mineral broths heals at 25 to 75 percent of the efficiency of water fasting, depending on the amount of nutrition taken and the amount the juices or broths are diluted. One would need to fast for a longer period to achieve the same results as a water fast.

If you decide to do a juice fast, note that most people can juice fast safely for up to 30 days, which is the typical norm. If you have hypoglycemia, diabetes, hypo thyroid, or Wilson's Syndrome, eat slices of avocado and banana every few hours (they digest slowly and maintain stable blood sugar levels), add high quality vegetable source protein powder to your juices, and add psyllium or other bulking agent to your juices twice a day to regulate blood sugar levels. Do not juice fast if you have impaired kidney function. Strain your juices and don't drink to bloating. The goal is to give the digestive system a rest. Anything solid, or with too many calories, activates the digestive process and delays the healing.

The Lemonade Fast
A good introductory juice fast is called the Lemonade Fast (See *The Master Cleanser* by Stanley Burroughs). A "lemonade" made with organic lemons, organic cayenne pepper, spring water, and organic Grade-B maple syrup is used to satisfy the body's cravings and mineral requirements while fasting.

The Salt Water Wash
Recommended by Burroughs as the start to the "lemonade fast," this is a good way to start any fast:

32 oz filtered water, 2 level teaspoons of non-iodized sea salt, mixed while warming for 30 seconds on a medium flame, drunk within 5 minutes; 1-3 hours later, it pushes (almost) everything out of your bowels.

Caloric Restriction

Even when not on an extended water or juice fast, you can still gain the benefits of a fast by reducing the number of meals per day. If, for example, you eat one main meal at 12 noon and then don't eat again until 12 noon the next day, you've effectively fasted for 24 hours, and have given your body a chance to rest and rejuvenate during that time. Caloric restriction is proven to extend life. This is beyond debate.

Enema during fasting?

Should you do an enema during a fast? I offer no definitive answer. Shelton advises against it as being unnecessary. Moser recommends it. My largest bowel movement came ten days into my fast upon performing a coffee enema! Now, I'm sure that movement would have occurred on its own in due time, but the peristaltic action of the bowel does slow considerably during a fast. And, since my sluggish bowel was what prompted me to start the fast, I used the enema to speed things along. That's my answer.

Benefits of Fasting

There are numerous benefits to fasting: Mental

clarity is improved and brain fog is lifted. Rapid, safe weight loss is achieved without flabbiness. The nervous system is balanced. Energy improves. The longer the fast, the greater an increase in energy and vitality. You may require less sleep. A thorough and deep detoxification occurs. Vital organs are rejuvenated. Your skin becomes even and softer. You have more mobility. You breathe more easily and more deeply. Digestion is more effective, and the peristaltic action of the intestines is stronger. Your taste buds are retrained to appreciate the flavors of real food.

Finally, fasting can raise your belief level about the control you have over your health and that health is not random. In other words, you become your own authority (Foundational Idea one). This final point is very critical. According to Moser and Solomon:

"...once a person has fasted long [often] enough to be certain of what their own body can do to fix itself, they acquire a degree of independence little known today. Many of those experienced with fasting no longer dread being without health insurance and feel far less need for a doctor or of having a regular checkup. They know with certainty that if something degenerates in their body, their own body can fix it by itself."----How and When to Be Your Own Doctor by Dr. Isabelle A. Moser with Steve Solomon

Download *The Stages of Fasting* infographic poster at:
www.agelessadept.com/resources

10. URINE THERAPY

What it is

Uropathy (*urine therapy, Amaroli*) is the ancient, proven and scientifically-supportable practice of ingesting small amounts of one's own urine, or of applying it topically as food, medicine, a restorative and transforming agent and immune system booster to heal a range of illnesses, including cancer.

Why it works

Despite our learned revulsion at the concept of ingesting our own urine, consider:

Urea (urine's "active" ingredient) has been used for decades in skin care/softening products.

You developed in amniotic fluid and your own urine for nine months before birth.

Now think about this from a different perspective. Let's recall from the FOUNDATION chapter:

Nature is perfect and foolproof.
The body is coded to heal.

Now, if you were designing a being with a foolproof strategy for self-healing that would allow access to the vital elements necessary for that healing, where would you put those elements? Would you put them all on trees and fruits that might only grow in certain regions and seasons? No. It would make more sense for each being to carry around his or her unique first aid kit right in their own bodies, wouldn't it?

And that's exactly how it is. Urine is a sterile, antiseptic fluid excreted by the kidneys. It is the excess nutrients, metabolites and water from the blood plasma that contains hormones, enzymes, vitamins, trace minerals and valuable biochemicals that are perfectly custom-tailored and unique to the current condition of the body that produces it. At this very moment, many companies are making millions extracting some of these substances from collected urine on a large scale.

But it's waste, isn't it? Again, let's take a look at Nature's logic. If it were that harmful to life and health, why design the body so it exits the body through the same region as life-creating sperm or through which a baby is born. Would that make sense?

Now, whether you agree with my speculative, philosophical arguments as to the logic of natural design, or not, the fact is that urine is not a waste product full of harmful substances as is commonly believed, but instead a treasure-trove of just the right bio-chemicals we need for our individual condition.

How to use it

<u>Morning urine</u>

Urine passed at any time of the day may be drunk

but the best urine is the mid-stream urine passed just after getting up in the morning. Collect it rejecting a little at the beginning and the end. Drink right away.

Topically/massage
Urine is used as a cleaner, skin tonic and to treat infections, wounds, and skin diseases.

Urine fast
Follow the directions for a water fast, and drink urine as well as water for the duration.

Universal Remedy
Mix 2 drops of urine in a tablespoon of pure water and shake. Keep in a dark dropper bottle and place a few drops under the tongue throughout the day. This is a homeopathic remedy that purports to cure all ills.

How it keeps the cells clean
Urine contains antibodies and immune stimulating factors against all viruses, harmful bacteria or fungi that we may harbor in our bodies. Researchers found that even minute amounts of antibodies, sometimes so low as to be undetectable with conventional methods, are effective in preventing and treating diseases.

For more, see:
The Water of Life by John Armstrong
Your Own Perfect Medicine by Martha Christy

11. BLOOD CLEANING

What it is

The habit of keeping the blood clean and toxin-free so it nourishes the body optimally and keeps your skin smooth and blemish-free.

How it keeps the cells clean

Herbs like burdock, echinacea, dandelion and black cohosh are blood cleansers. Many bumps, carbuncles, blemishes and growths on the skin are caused by impure blood coursing through your body. In fact, almost any blemish can and should be cleaned from the inside. If you insist on applying topical creams and ointments without addressing the cause, you'll be covering and masking them with harmful chemicals for the rest of your days. If you clean your skin from the inside and maintain the clean cell lifestyle, you only have to do it once.

How to do it

Drink herbal teas; sprinkle herbs in powdered form into your juices and smoothies; take echinacea, dandelion or other herbal combination supplements.

12. OIL PULLING

What it is

Oil pulling (an Ayurvedic practice) is an oral detoxification procedure done by swishing a tablespoon of oil (sesame, coconut, olive) in your mouth for 10-20 minutes.

How it keeps the cells clean

Oil pulling works by cleaning the oral cavity in a similar way that soap cleans dirty dishes. It sucks out the (toxins) creating a clean, antiseptic oral environment needed to prevent cavities and disease. However, its benefits go further and has been used to treat tooth decay, bad breath, bleeding gums, heart disease, inflammation, as well as whiten teeth, prevent cavities, improve acne and boost the immune system.

How to do it

• Upon rising, before brushing teeth or drinking:

• Gently swish 1 – 2 tablespoons of coconut oil in your mouth and between teeth for 10-20 minutes. Don't swallow any of the oil.

• Spit out the oil in the trash or toilet (not the sink).

• Rinse with warm salt water or GSE water.

CHAPTER 7: Cleaners ▲

In conjunction with the practices in the previous section, the following naturally-occurring substances help in maintaining a clean cell body:

Elements, minerals (sulfur, oxygen, silver...)

1. MMS
2. Hydrogen Peroxide
3. DMSO
4. Colloidal Silver

Plant-based extracts/oils

5. Olive Leaf Extract
6. Grapefruit Seed Extract
7. Tea Tree Oil
8. Oil of Oregano

Earth-based

9. Clay
10. Diatomaceous Earth

MMS

Miracle Mineral Solution

What it is

When Sodium Chlorite solution ($NaClO_2$) is combined with a 50% solution of citric acid, a chemical reaction takes place within the resulting solution. A man named Jim Humble called that solution Miracle Mineral Solution, when in 1996, he used an early version of it to completely cure four members of his mining crew who had malaria. The gas produced, Chlorine Dioxide (CLO_2) is a curative agent with some almost miraculous healing properties.

How it keeps the cells clean

CLO_2 is a powerful disinfectant that can be used to eliminate worms, purify water, treat malaria and a wide range of illnesses.

How to use it

You'll typically purchase a bottle of sodium chlorite and a bottle of citric acid. Combine in 1:1 ratio, let sit for 30 seconds to allow reaction. Then add to juice or water and drink. You can also use MMS solution as body wash, enema or intestinal cleanser.

Read more at: www. jimhumble.co

HYDROGEN PEROXIDE (H2O2)

What it is

FOOD GRADE hydrogen peroxide, not your supermarket or pharmacy peroxide.

How it keeps the cells clean

H2O2 therapy has been used successfully for: allergies, altitude sickness, Alzheimer's, anemia, arrhythmia asthma, bacterial infections, bronchitis, cancer, candida, cardiovascular disease, cerebral vascular disease, chronic pain, prostatitis, diabetes Type II, diabetic gangrene, diabetic retinopathy, Epstein-Barr, emphysema, food allergies, fungal infections, gingivitis, Herpes Simplex, Herpes Zoster, HIV Infection, influenza, insect bites, liver cirrhosis, Lupus Erythematosis, Multiple Sclerosis, parasitic infections, Parkinsonism, gum disease, rheumatoid arthritis, shingles, sinusitis, sore throat, ulcers, viral infections, warts and yeast infections.

Hydrogen peroxide is an extremely powerful cleanser for the blood and digestive tract. If your system is very toxic, you may experience a healing crisis--fatigue, diarrhea, headaches, skin eruptions, cold or flu-like symptoms, and nausea. If so, do not discontinue the therapy. Go back to a lower number of drops until the symptoms ease, then resume.

Hydrogen Peroxide cleansing schedule

Food grade hydrogen peroxide (H2O2) is available in different strengths online and at health food stores. This chart shows the number of drops to use as a cleansing regimen for three concentrations. Take on an empty stomach, 1 hour before meals or 3 hours after. If taken too close to meals, it may react with bacteria in the food, causing foaming, indigestion and even vomiting. Avoid taking too close to bedtime as it can energize you and result in sleeplessness.

Day #	3%	12%	35%	Times per day
1	20 drops	6 drops	2 drops	3
2	40 drops	12 drops	4 drops	3
3	60 drops	18 drops	6 drops	3
4	80 drops	24 drops	8 drops	3
5	100 drops	30 drops	10 drops	3
6	120 drops	36 drops	12 drops	3
7	140 drops	42 drops	14 drops	3
8	160 drops	48 drops	16 drops	3
9	180 drops	54 drops	18 drops	3
10	200 drops	60 drops	20 drops	3
11	200 drops	60 drops	20 drops	3
12	200 drops	60 drops	20 drops	3
13	200 drops	60 drops	20 drops	3
14	200 drops	60 drops	20 drops	3
15	200 drops	60 drops	20 drops	3
16	200 drops	60 drops	20 drops	3

DMSO

What it is

DMSO, or dimethyl sulfoxide, is a by-product of papermaking. It is a colorless industrial solvent first identified in 1866 by a Russian scientist.

What it does to keep the cells clean

DMSO provides rapid relief of pain, increased mobility and reduction of inflammation when used topically (on the skin).

Given soon after a stroke, DMSO can dissolve the clot that causes the stroke, restoring circulation and avoiding paralysis.

DMSO may help neutralize harmful effects to the heart and brain from medical disorders involving the head and spinal chord injury, stroke, memory dysfunction, and ischemic heart disease.

DMSO can dissolve a virus' protein coating, leaving the virus core unprotected with its nucleic acid exposed to the immune system. Applied topically, it alleviates the lesions that occur as a result of Herpes Zoster (shingles).

DMSO can be effective in the treatment of painful corns, calluses, ingrown toenails, bunions, hammertoes, heel spurs, and the inflammation of gouty big toes.

Uses for specific conditions

A concentration of 50% to 80% applied two or three times a day will flatten a raised scar after several months.

One drop of a 25% DMSO solution (diluted in sterile physiologic or saline solution) once or twice per day is useful for eye problems, including cataracts or glaucoma.

Because DMSO permeates the skin, one of its main uses is to transport other substances more deeply into the body. For instance, mixing DMSO with tea tree oil and applying it to toenail fungus transmits the tea tree oil more deeply to eliminate the condition. This also means one should take caution when handling DMSO and make sure one's hands are clean so as not to transport harmful chemicals into the body.

More:
www.sott.net/article/228453-DMSO-The-Real-Miracle-Solution

https://web.archive.org/web/20110405102312/http://www.livestr ong.com/article/175630-benefits-of-dmso

COLLOIDAL SILVER

What it is

Colloidal silver is a suspension of submicroscopic metallic silver particles in water. It is made by sending a small electrical current to two silver electrodes placed in distilled water. The water becomes flooded with tiny nanoparticles of silver.

How it keeps the cells clean

• is alkaline, kills bacteria; a natural antibiotic; known as a second immune system. Silver's negative ions binds with pathogens' positive ions.

• kills 650 organisms; helps destroy bacteria, fungi and viruses; (antibiotics are effective only against about 12 forms of bacteria and fungi, but never viruses.)

• is helpful for acne, allergies, arthritis, athlete's foot, boils, burns, Candida, cystitis, diabetes, eczema and hay fever.

• is helpful against indigestion, parasitic infections, psoriasis, ringworm, warts and yeast infections; acne, AIDS, allergies, appendicitis, arthritis, athlete's foot, bladder inflammation, blood parasites, blood poisoning, boils, bums, cancer, cholera, colitis, conjunctivitis, cystitis, dermatitis, diabetes, dysentery, eczema, fibrositis, gastritis, gonorrhoea, hay fever, herpes, impetigo, indigestion, keratitis, leprosy, leukemia, lupus, lymphangitis, Lyme disease, meningitis, neurasthenia, parasitic infections: viral, fungal and bacterial pneumonia, pleurisy, prostate pruritus ani, psoriasis, purulent opthalmia, rhinitis, rheumatism, ringworm, scarlet fever, septic conditions of the eyes, ears, mouth, and throat seborrhea, septic~ shingles, skin cancer, staphylococcus and streptococcus infections, stomach flu, syphilis, thyroid, tuberculosis, tonsillitis, toxemia, trachoma, all forms of virus, warts, whooping cough, yeast infection, stomach ulcer, canine parovirus plus fungal and viral attacks on plants.

How to use it

Swishing the solution under the tongue briefly before swallowing ensures fast absorption. In three to four days the silver will accumulate in the tissues sufficiently for benefits to begin. Since colloidal silver is eliminated by the kidneys, lymph system and bowels after three weeks, a regular daily intake is recommended to protect against dangerous pathogens. You can purchase your own colloidal silver maker and make batches for pennies.[See Resources]

OLIVE LEAF EXTRACT (OLE)

What it is

Olive Leaf Extract is the dried, ground leaves of the olive tree in capsule or tea form.

How it keeps the cells clean

Olive Leaf Extract is astringent, anti-bacterial, antifungal, anti-oxidant, anti-parasitic, anti-septic, antiviral, febrifuge, immune-booster and tranquilizer used to treat parasites (giardia, intestinal worms, protozoa, pinworms, ringworm, roundworm, tapeworms), infection, arthritis, autoimmune disorders, chlamydia, chronic fatigue, chronic joint ache, toenail fungus infection, colds & flu, cold sores, dengue, EpsteinBarr virus, fibromyalgia, gastric ulcers caused by H. pylori, genital herpes, genital warts, gonorrhea pain, hepatitis A, B, C, herpes I and II, HIV / ARC / AIDS, human herpes virus 6, 7, lupus, malaria, bacterial/viral meningitis, mononucleosis, staphylococcal food poisoning, streptococcus throat infection, syphilis, toothache, trichinosis, vaginitis and tuberculosis.

How to use it

Look for brands with at least 25% oleuropein content. Follow directions in capsule, tea bag, tincture and bulk powder forms. May be used as skin wash.

GRAPEFRUIT SEED EXTRACT (GSE)

What it is

As the name accurately implies, GSE is the bitter, concentrated extract made from grapefruit seeds.

How it keeps the cells clean

GSE has been shown to be effective in treating hundreds of different organisms including: Shigella, Staphylococcus, Pseudomonas aeruginosa, Giardia lamblia, Diplococcus pneumoniae, Haemophilus influenzae, Mycobacterium species, Campylobacter, Candida albicans, Escherichia coli, Streptococcus, Salmonella, Klebsiella, Proteus, Cholera, Chlamydia trachomatis, Trichomonas vaginalis, Legionella pneumoniae, Helicobacter pylori, Herpes simplex 1, Influenza A2, and measles virus. It has been shown to kill both gram-negative and gram-positive bacteria.

Internal uses include, but are not limited to: digestive upsets, gastrointestinal disorders, diarrhea and food poisoning; infections from parasites (single and multi-celled), bacteria, viruses and fungus; candida yeast infections, thrush and chronic fatigue. It is good for oral infections including tooth plaque, gum disorders, and bad breath; colds and flu, sore throats, strep throat, ear inflammation, pain, bloating, sinusitis and other ailments.

External uses include, but are not limited to: acne,

athlete's foot, nail fungus infections, skin infections caused by fungus, bacteria, parasites, viruses, ringworm, cuts and wounds, warts, poison ivy, poison oak, rashes, jock itch, shaving itch, dandruff, cold sores, head lice, chickenpox, cracked lips and more.

Physicians have observed that the herpes simplex virus becomes inactive just ten minutes after the application of grapefruit seed extract.

GSE properties

Broad Spectrum

Grapefruit seed extract's main advantage is it's extraordinary ability to perform internally and externally against a wide variety of infections caused by viruses, bacteria, fungi and parasites.

Alkalizing

Grapefruit seed extract helps alkalize the body. It is considered one of the most alkaline forming substances and the fruit is very alkalizing. Alkalizing the body (raising pH) is one of the single most important health regeneration benefits available. Disease cannot live in an alkaline environment within the body. It is claimed that cancer dies in a pH of 8.0. Countless other conditions are caused by an acid environment within the body. These same conditions are effectively treated by restoring the proper pH. Even though grapefruit seed extract's pH is a low 2.0, acid foods have alkaline effects on the body. Alkaline foods like meat, sugar and most grains create an acid environment within the body. Most degenerative diseases are associated with your body pH, and is one of the most important aspects to consider when trying to overcome a serious illness and maintain good health. Many diseases are caused from improper pH.

Promotes Beneficial Bacteria
Grapefruit seed extract stimulates the immune system. According to doctors and veterinarians, grapefruit seed extract at normal doses is gentle yet preserves the integrity of your intestinal bacteria.

Effective against drug-resistant bacteria
To date there is no evidence that any type of pathogenic microorganism has ever built up a resistance to grapefruit seed extract's active ingredient. Due to the mode of its activity, it is believed that this resistance is impossible as grapefruit seed extract disrupts the organisms cytoplasmic membrane.

Non-toxic
GSE can be taken for long periods without toxic side effects. There are reports that people have taken grapefruit seed extract every day for several years (as a preventive) without side effects of any kind.

Hypoallergenic (non-allergenic)

Dr. Allen Sachs points out that about 3 to 5 percent of all people are allergic to citrus fruit and could therefore also display a sensitive reaction to grapefruit seed extract. These people should start with a low dosage and perform a patch test to be sure.

Economical & long-lasting

GSE has a long shelf life (years) and is effective at low concentrations. Most applications require just a few drops per dose. A 1.5oz bottle yields 900 drops.

GSE uses

Safe for animals (pets, fish, reptiles, birds etc).

Animals benefit from the use of grapefruit extract for internal and external conditions and infections, skin conditions, mange, fleas, etc.

A household disinfectant and garden cleaner

Use as a vegetable wash, for counter tops and cutting boards. Use as a tool cleaner to remove fungus or mold, or as a bug or plant spray. Use in laundry rinse cycle to eliminate fungus and bacteria. It is more effective at killing germs than alcohol or surgical soap. *Tip: I keep a "GSE spray bottle" handy (5-8 drops in 16-24 ounces of purified water) and use for disinfecting cutting boards, kitchen/bathroom surfaces, and drink or gargle with it during the day.*

<u>A traveler's first aid mainstay</u>

Can be used to protect against water and food borne illnesses, diarrhea, dysentery, etc.

<u>Wound Healing</u>

Extremely good for fast healing of scar tissue associated with many types of wounds.

GSE dosages for specific conditions
(these doses apply to regular strength GSE)

Acne - Add a few drops to skin care products. Avoid contact with eyes. After cleansing the face, apply 2 to 3 drops of GSE to moistened fingertips, and massage gently in circular motions for one minute. Rinse with cool water. The bacteria-killing properties and cleansing action may cause a tingling sensation.

AIDS - An increasing number of HIV positive people are able to improve their immune system by using GSE to fight viruses, bacteria, fungi, Candida, or parasites. It's best to start with a diluted concentration, so the body can adjust to the detoxification process.

Athlete's foot - The commercially prepared foot powders, creams, and sprays that contain GSE have been shown to be beneficial for athlete's foot.

Colds, flu, viruses - Take 10 - 15 drops, or 1 - 2 capsules/tablets, 3 times a day, at the first signs of cold or flu. Or mix 50 drops in 1 quart of juice, and sip throughout the day.

Chronic Fatigue Syndrome - To generally build up immune system, gradually increase GSE amount to the recommended dosage for colds, flu, and viruses.

Cold sores, cuts, wounds - Use 1 - 5 drops in 50 drops of water. Frequent application of solution to wound will promote faster healing.

Gums (Gingivitis) - Dilute 5 to 10 drops of GSE in 6 to 8 ounces of water, and rinse mouth thoroughly.

Dandruff - Add a few drops to each application of shampoo. Wait 5 minutes. Rinse. Avoid eyes.

Diarrhea - Use 15 to 20 drops in juice every four hours; no more than 60 drops per day. For parasites, higher doses may be necessary.

Earaches - Commercially prepared eardrops containing GSE can be found at the health food stores. Do not use GSE concentrate directly in ears.

Parasites - 3 to 5 doses per day. Parasite infections that have occurred for a long period of time will take more time to cure. Be patient.

Respiratory infections - Use in nebulizers (1 drop GSE to one ounce saline water).

Sinusitis - Using a spray atomizer, add a pinch of salt, and no more than two drops of GSE. Shake and spray into nose. Repeat every four hours. If the solution is too mild, add one or two more drops of GSE and shake. Do not use with young children.

Sore throats - Dilute a few drops in water and use as a gargle. This will fight even Strep germs. Use 2 to 3 drops in 5 ounces of water for the gargle.

Traveler's Diarrhea - Use 1 - 2 drops of GSE in a glass of water each day as a preventive.

Ulcers - Use 2-3 drops in 12 ounces of juice or water, and take with one meal. If no stomach irritation occurs, increase to two, and then three meals per day.

Other Uses
Water purification - Add 10 to 25 drops of GSE, per gallon of water. Shake and let stand for several minutes. The water will have a bitter taste to it.

Cleaning produce - Add a few drops to water used for washing produce. Let sit for 5 to 10 minutes. Rinse thoroughly. Destroys Salmonella/E.Coli bacteria. It's the active ingredient in most brands of vegetable wash.

Pet health - GSE is a remedy for skin disease, external injuries, fungal infections, parasites, bacteria, and viruses. Helps bad breath added to drinking water. Use 1 drop per 10 pounds of animal body weight.

Carpet cleaner - Use to kill Staphylococcus, Streptococcus, Salmonella and other pathogens.

Pools - Use in hot tubs and pools; less chlorine.

Humidifiers - (3 - 4 drops per gallon of water) to prevent algae growth in any stagnant water.

Preservative - instead of chemical preservatives.

Animal feed - Add to animal feed and water to reduce the incidence of infectious diseases.

Note: grapefruit juice is known to increase the absorption rate of certain pharmaceuticals. Check with your pharmacist or doctor if on medication.

TEA TREE OIL

What it is

Tea tree oil (TTO), also called melaleuca oil, is made from the leaves of the tea tree plant (Melaleuca alternifolia), which is native to Australia.

How it keeps the cells clean

Tea tree oil is antibacterial, antimicrobial, antiseptic, antiviral, balsamic, cicatrisant, expectorant, fungicide and an insecticide. It treats acne, relieves rashes and other skin conditions (eczema, warts), prevents lice, cures toenail fungus, freshens breath, treats warts, sanitizes cuts, and is an all-purpose household cleaner. It provides relief from cough, colds, bronchitis and congestion, cures viral infections and boosts the immune system. Steam inhalation clears congested nasal passages and kills bacteria.

How to use it

Apply topically. Do not swallow. Do not use full strength. For skin conditions, mix 1 tablespoon of a "carrier oil" (olive, jojoba, coconut) with 8-10 drops of tea tree oil and apply to irritated areas. For sinus conditions, add a few drops to a steaming bowl of purified water, cover head with towel and inhale vapors for five to ten minutes.

OIL OF OREGANO

What it is

Oil of oregano is oil from the leaves and flowers of *Origanum vulgare*, native to the Mediterranean, or *Thymus capitatus* (Spain)--not your kitchen oregano.

How it keeps the cells clean

Oil of oregano is an antiviral, antibacterial, antifungal agent rivaling pharmaceutical antibiotics such as streptomycin, penicillin, vacnomycin, nystatin, and amphotericin in its ability to eliminate microbes. It destroys organisms that contribute to skin infections and digestive problems; strengthens the immune system; increases joint and muscle flexibility; improves respiratory health and sinus conditions; stops infections (cold/ flu); fights yeast and fungi; helps with allergies and hay fever; helps gum/mouth conditions, burns, wounds, cuts and sore muscles.

How to use it

Place a few drops under the tongue once or twice a day or at the first feeling of a "cold" or to address specific issues listed above. Mix a few drops with orange juice to mask the taste.

CLAY

What it is

Clay is earth. Each type (red clay, French green clay, bentonite), offers unique benefits. I also place Diatomaceous Earth in this category.

How it keeps the cells clean

Clay's minerals are negatively charged while toxins tend to be positively charged. Therefore, they attract and bind with each other.

Benefits reported by people using liquid clay for a period of two to four weeks include: improved intestinal regularity; relief from chronic constipation, diarrhea, indigestion, and ulcers; a surge in physical energy; clearer complexion; brighter, whiter eyes; enhanced alertness; emotional uplift; improved tissue and gum repair; and increased resistance to infections.

Clay:

• Detoxifies the digestive system (the adsorptive action of clay pulls contaminants from the body)

• Fights bacterial, organic and non-organic toxicity

• Eliminates internal parasites (digestive tract)

• Provides immune system support (used internally, stimulates elimination and supports organ function)

• Fixes free oxygen in the blood stream (occurs once the liver has been restored to full function)

• Increases T-cell count

- Fights free radicals
- Combats mercury poisoning
- Acts as a trace mineral supplement
- Aids liver detoxification
- Helps stomach aches and bacterial food poisoning
- Acts as an alkalizing agent in the body

Uses for specific conditions

Bone and Muscle Damage due to Traumatic Injury

Apply clay pack immediately after injury; applied 1/2 - 1 inch thick and covered, changed as needed (1/2 - 12 hrs.), duration to maximum tolerance.

Carpal Tunnel Syndrome, Tendinitis

Apply clay wrap around entire area if possible, 1/4 1/2 inch thick, covered, for 20 minutes to an hour initially, increased to overnight as tolerance permits, for three days to three weeks.

Treatment of Internal Organs

Apply clay compress (dressing saturated with hydrated clay) to area for 20 minutes per application to start. Extend to 1 hour as tolerable, progress to clay pack and 20 minute treatments, then to one hour.

Chronic Headaches

Apply clay pack to nape of the neck for twenty minutes, then apply to the forehead for twenty minutes (continue to alternate as needed).

Skin Conditions (acne, eczema, rashes, more)

Depending on the condition, clay compresses or packs can be used (any cystic condition requires dense packs applied for an extended amount of time).

Rapid healing of injuries (bruises, sprains, burns, etc.)

Apply thick clay packs to sprains, bruises, breaks, etc. Apply thin clay strips, covered, or compressed to burns. For any injury that includes a break in the skin, never allow the clay to dry. Re-dress as needed.

Severe Bacterial Infections

Clean wound thoroughly with liquid bentonite; Apply clay packs of at least 1/2 inch thick. Change dressings as often as required due to drainage. Never allow clay to dry on damaged tissues.

Skin rejuvenation and deep cleansing

One to twelve cups of bentonite added to a hot bath; hydrated bentonite used as a normal soap; clay masks applied to the skin; clay formulations used in a massage treatment.

DIATOMACEOUS EARTH (DE)

What it is

Food grade Diatomaceous Earth (DE) is an allnatural off-white "dirt" made from the tiny fossilized remains of marine phytoplankton/water plants. DE contains silica, a vital nutrient for the body's functions.

How it keeps the cells clean

Silica (in collagen) benefits the hair, skin, nails, teeth and gums. It stimulates the immune system, promotes healthy cholesterol levels, increased metabolism for energy, lung tissue elasticity, lymph nodes, urinary tract, reduced inflammation in intestines; it may strengthen blood vessels, normalize blood pressure, hemorrhoids, decrease vertigo, tinnitus and insomnia and help joints and rheumatism. Silica may alleviate Alzheimer's disease by preventing the body from absorbing aluminum and by flushing aluminum from the tissues. Similar to clay, it's unique physical structure and negative charge attracts and absorbs fungi, protozoa, viruses, endotoxins, pesticides, drug residues, E.coli, and heavy metals.

How to use it

Simply mix one to two teaspoons of this off-white dirt in your juice, smoothies or in plain water.

SECTION III

CHAPTER 8: Nutrients ▲

Why to eat?

Just as Carrel did, to keep our cells alive, we must also focus on introducing nutrients to the body. Before we do so, however, here's a question: What's the purpose of food? It may seem silly to ask, but why do you or any of us eat? To stay alive? Sure, (although Breatharians might disagree), but beyond that?

It can't always be about comfort.
"In our society, we've been sold a childish belief that we can continue our destructive behaviors, yet expect to reap creative benefits. We want to taste the sugar, but not experience its effects. We want to live in excess, without the accumulation. We then place our hopes in magic pills or potions that will wipe away the effects of our actions."
— from *The Man Who Lived Forever*

For many people, eating is simply one of life's pleasures--a social activity strictly for the taste buds.

I'd like to suggest, however, that you think of eating as much more. You eat to survive. You eat to bring nutrition into the body. You should also eat to cleanse. You should also eat to heal and rejuvenate and reverse aging. Part of the requirement for healthy living and reversing the aging process is that you be willing, eager and even happy to eat foods that don't particularly taste good in order to reap their benefits. You must be willing to take a few drops of the extremely bitter grapefruit seed extract, a few burning drops of oil of oregano, a capful of vile-tasting wood root tonic or bitters, or some of your least favorite vegetables in order to assist your body in reclaiming and maintaining its youth. This is not to say that reversing the aging process through the Clean Cell Protocol is difficult, unappetizing or distasteful. I've prepared meals for friends and family that have called their own cooking into question, and have far surpassed their expectations of what they think a "healthy" meal tastes like. However, it simply means that your taste for some of the things I'll suggest may need to be "acquired."

What to eat

In a simpler, pristine world, you could achieve optimal nutrition with this simple rule: *"eat real food in as close to its natural, living state as possible."*

Unfortunately, however, nutrition is not the default setting of the standard western diet. Nutrition won't just happen as a function of eating. Nutrition is no longer simply a function of the food we eat but also of the soil in which it is grown, how long it remains nourished by the tree/vine/soil, how it is prepared, chewed, digested and even how it is eliminated. These factors have all been adversely affected by capitalism, advertising, societal habits and belief systems. You need to be deliberate about it. The new rules are:

• Eat food in as close to its natural state as possible; Nothing processed. Nothing "refined." Nothing fried. Nothing homogenized or pasteurized or microwaved.
• Eat raw fruits, vegetables, nuts, seeds when possible. (Don't kill food by cooking.)
• Go organic, supplement with superfoods.
• Add a bit of cayenne and ginger to aid digestion.
• Eat more sprouts and seaweeds.
• Pick your own fruits; grow your own vegetables

Why raw?

Raw food is living food with enzymes and higher concentrations of MSM.

Why nothing microwaved?

Microwaves alter food's molecular structure.

When to eat

Eat your main meal between noon and 3pm when your body's energy is at its peak and to allow time for proper digestion and elimination before you sleep. Eat only when hungry. Drink liquids about 1-2 hours after eating. Drinking while eating dilutes the strength of the stomach acids and causes poor digestion.

A BASIC FOOD LIST

Since everyone's exposure to and awareness of food options vary widely, here are some foods, concepts, supplements and preparation tips to help improve the quality, taste and nutritional benefit of the food you prepare for yourself and those you love.

To drink

Drink rain water, spring water, coconut water, fresh-squeezed fruit juices and nectars, lemonade sweetened with maple syrup, bottled water, distilled water (for making colloidal silver).

Probiotics

Probiotic foods help keep the colon's digestive and eliminative process functioning optimally. This includes kimchee, cultured vegetables, miso, soy yogurt and other fermented foods.

Sprouts

You can and should grow your own sprouts. You can have a tray or sprouting bottle of sprouted lentils, beans of all sorts on your counter top ready to add to salads or to eat directly.

Grains

Quinoa

One of few alkaline "grains." Good source of complete protein ("incomplete" grains lack the amino acids lysine and isoleucine); provides manganese, phosphorus, copper, magnesium, fiber, folate, zinc, phytonutrients; is anti-inflammatory; decreases risk of diabetes, and, is actually not a grain, but is in the same family as spinach, Swiss chard and beets.

Millet

Provides copper, phosphorus, manganese and magnesium which reduces the severity of asthma, the frequency of migraine attacks, lowers high blood pressure and reduces the risk of heart attack; protects against heart disease, gallstones, breast cancer; plus tastes great with pumpkin seed oil or olive oil on top!

Brown rice

Provides manganese, selenium, phosphorus, copper, magnesium, iron and vitamins B1, B3 & B6. The milling and polishing inflicted upon brown rice to make it white, destroys 50% of the manganese, 50% of the phosphorus, 60% of the iron, 80% of the vitamin B1, 67% of the vitamin B3, 90% of the vitamin B6, and all the dietary fiber and essential fatty acids. Brown rice is better for you. This is beyond debate.

Barley

Provides molybdenum, manganese, fiber, selenium, copper, vitamin B1, chromium, phosphorus, magnesium, vitamin B3 and fiber for enhanced bowel function; lowers cholesterol; promotes good intestinal flora; lowers risk of type 2 Diabetes, and tastes great with spirulina and your favorite oil on top!

Oils

"Smoke point" is the temperature at which enough volatile compounds emerge from oil that a bluish smoke becomes clearly visible. Avocado oil has one of the highest smoke points, which makes it great for cooking. However, the best indicator of how good an oil is for cooking is its saturated fat content. While many argue that saturated fat content is bad for you, a higher value means the oil does not break down into harmful, cancer causing compounds when used for cooking. So, though other oils have higher smoke points, coconut oil is one of the most stable for frying.

Oil	Smoke point	Saturated fat
avocado oil	520°F (270°C)	12.10%
sunflower oil	440°F (226°C)	10.79%
Grapeseed oil	420°F (216°C)	10.00%
olive oil (Extra virgin)	375°F (190°C)	14.19%
corn oil	352°F (178°)	13.60%
coconut oil (virgin)	350°F (177°C)	91.92%
sesame oil (unrefined)	350°F (177°C)	14.85%
flax seed oil	225°F (107°C)	9.40%

Coconut oil
Promotes strong bones, weight loss and healthy hair; regulates digestion; enhances immunity, energy and mineral absorption; fights bacteria, fungi and viruses; very stable at high temperatures, so is best oil for cooking; use for oil pulling, skin rejuvenation, sunblock and as a daily supplement.

Olive oil
Provides unsaturated fat, omega-3 fatty acids; balances cholesterol levels; reduces inflammation; prevents heart disease and prostate tumors; lowers blood sugar; moisturizes skin. Use on salads, on rice or grains, or as daily supplement, but not for cooking.

Grapeseed oil
Great for cooking, grapeseed oil is also one of the best oils for massages because of its texture.

Flax seed oil
First cultivated in Europe; source of Omega oils (3&6); promotes fertility and heart health; eases constipation, inflammation, gallstones and nerve damage; contains lignans which regulate hormones; helps the prostate, infertility and impotence; not for cooking. Use on rice and salads; take orally daily. Ground seeds make a good flour and provide fiber to relieve constipation.

Pumpkin seed oil

Pumpkin seeds, pumpkin seed extracts, and pumpkin seed oil are well known for their antimicrobial benefits, including anti-fungal and anti-viral properties. Doesn't sound appetizing, but you'll forget about the clinical-sounding benefits once you taste it! Try pouring over cooked grains like millet!

Sesame oil

Provides copper, manganese, calcium, phosphorus, magnesium, iron, zinc, molybdenum, vitamin B1, selenium and fiber; eases arthritis pain; promotes bone/joint strength; lowers blood pressure; prevents colon cancer, osteoporosis, migraines and lowers cholesterol. Recommended for oil pulling in most texts, but coconut oil is equally effective.

Black seed oil

For thousands of years, people in Asia, Africa, the Middle East and the Mediterranean, used black seed (Nigella Sativa) for asthma, backache, diabetes, diarrhea, nasal congestion, graying hair, hair loss, hay fever, headaches and to promote well being; eases hypertension, fatigue, muscular pain, toothaches and ulcers; supports mental function and sexual potency. I put a teaspoon in my "Comeback Cocktale" as a daily tonic. (See Resource List for Bionatal® discount code)

Seaweed
Irish moss
Aka "carrageen moss" (Scientific names: *Chondrus crispus* or *Gracilaria*). Mineral-rich, it is boiled with cinnamon and milk to make a thick drink for male virility both in Trinidad & Tobago, as well as in Jamaica—where the drink is called "Put it Back!" Use in smoothies, soups and porridge.

Kelp
Provides iodine for efficient thyroid and pituitary function, iron, calcium, potassium and magnesium; promotes weight loss and nail/hair growth; enhances the immune system; fights off infection. Include in soups, salads. Add last to dishes.

Other sea weeds
Other sea weeds include dulse, hiziki and kombuka. I use seaweeds liberally in all my dishes; sprinkle kelp or dulse on stir-fries or mix into salads.

Sweeteners
Maple syrup
Use to sweeten instead of sugar. Contains fewer calories and more minerals than honey. Provides calcium, chromium, copper, iron, magnesium, manganese, phosphorus, potassium, selenium, sodium and zinc. Use mineral-rich Grade B in lemonade fast.

Blackstrap molasses

This dark liquid byproduct of the process of refining sugar cane is the concentrated substance left over after the sugar's sucrose has been crystallized. Contains manganese, copper, iron, calcium, potassium, magnesium, vitamin B6 (pyridoxine), and selenium. Provides the minerals for reducing graying hair.

Honey

Raw Manuka honey fights infection and aids tissue healing; reduces inflammation and scarring; treats diarrhea, indigestion, ulcers and gastroenteritis.

Superfoods

Apple cider vinegar

Promotes stamina; regulates cholesterol and metabolism; enhances immune system and digestion; cures skin conditions, acne, constipation, arthritis and gout; fights allergies, urinary tract infections and food poisoning; use in salads.

Barley grass powder

Extremely alkaline; concentrated source of minerals, amino acids and vitamins including B12; inhibits cancer including prostate, leukemia and brain tumors; promotes digestion, age reversal, heart health and weight loss; eases arthritis and ulcers;.

Garlic
Natural antibiotic and immune enhancer. Garlic's allicin increases blood flow. Add raw to salads, add last to stir fries and soups.

Bee pollen
This is one of Nature's most complete foods. Richest known source of vitamins, minerals, amino acids, hormones, enzymes and fats; natural antibiotic; promotes growth of healthy new cells, tissue repair, toxin elimination, resistance to infections, fertility in women and calmness. Regulates cholesterol levels, blood pressure and nervous system. Enhances sexual activity, memory, stamina and endurance. Combats cancer, diabetes, arthritis and depression. Use in cereal, yogurt and smoothies.

Chlorella powder
Highest amount of chlorophyll of any plant; balances cholesterol; promotes good bacteria and energy; enhances digestion; eases constipation, ulcers and colitis; fights infection, radiation; treats fibromyalgia, cancer and radiation exposure; 60% protein, 18 amino acids and B12; use in green juices.

Goji berries
Also called "wolfberry"; used in Asia for over 6000 years; promotes longevity; enhances immune

function; fights cancer; increases fertility and male sexual function by improving circulation. Sprinkle on cereals. Use as tea. Add to smoothies.

Lecithin
(available as soy lecithin)
Promotes cell permeability; regulates good/bad cholesterol; balances circulatory and nervous systems; reverses heart disease; enhances brain/memory function; fights atherosclerosis; repairs liver damage due to alcohol. Use on salads.

Nutritional yeast
Provides B vitamins (sometimes B12), trace minerals, protein and all 18 amino acids; enhances energy and memory; free of dairy, soy, gluten, sugar and animal products; will not aggravate Candida. Sprinkle on salads, popcorn, rice and quinoa.

Maca powder
Cultivated in Peru as an aphrodisiac for over 3000 years; increases energy; improves fertility; regulates hormones; reduces depression; enhances mental clarity; reduces anxiety; improves circulation; builds muscle; improves skin tone; promotes hair growth and thyroid function; increases libido/sexual function in men and women. Use in smoothies and shakes; sprinkle on fruit. Use in CockTale (see Recipes).

Malunggay

Aka *Moringa Oleifera*; provides 90+ vitamins, minerals and phytonutrients, over 46 antioxidants and 36 anti-inflammatory compounds. 7 times the vitamin C of oranges, 4 times the vitamin A of carrots, 4 times the calcium of milk, 3 times the potassium of bananas and 2 times the protein of yogurt; contains 18 amino acids, including eight essential ones.

Pumpkin seeds

Discovered in Mexican caves dating 7,000 BC, and used in ancient Greece; provides copper, iron, manganese, magnesium, phosphorus and protein; lowers cholesterol levels; prevents osteoporosis and kidney stones; fights prostate cancer; combats tapeworms, parasites and arthritis; one of the best natural sources of zinc. Use in smoothies, grind and add to coleslaw.

Royal jelly

Provides vitamins, minerals, proteins and antioxidants; boosts strength and energy; promotes hormonal balance in men and women; enhances concentration and brain function; fights insomnia; repairs bones, nails and hair; combats impotence and frigidity; improves endurance, resistance to viruses and bacteria; restores appetite; stimulates libido.

Spirulina

Spirulina is perhaps the most nutritionally complete of all food supplements; provides protein, complex carbohydrates, iron, vitamins A, K, and B complex, beta carotene and antioxidants; rich in chlorophyll, lipids, fatty nucleic acids, iron, magnesium, trace minerals, B12 and gamma-linolenic acid (a compound in breast milk); promotes digestion and bowel function; enhances eyesight; builds muscle; increases stamina; stimulates intestinal flora; combats cellular degeneration and radiation sickness; improves absorption; reduces bad cholesterol; provides 8 essential/10 non-essential amino acids plus zinc; detoxifies blood. Use in salads, juices, smoothies, shakes; sprinkle on rice and grains.

The following two charts will show just how nutritionally superior these super foods are.

Superfood Nutrient Comparison

Nutrient	Moringa	Bee Pollen	Spirulina	Chlorella
Vitamin A (Beta Carotene)	√	√	√	√
Vitamin B1 (Thiamine)	√	√	√	√
Vitamin B2	√	√	√	√
Vitamin B3 (Niacin)	√	√	√	√
Vitamin B5 (Pantothenic Acid)		√	√	√
Vitamin B6 (Pyridoxine)	√	√	√	√
Vitamin B12		√	√	√
Vitamin C (Ascorbic Acid)	√	√	√	√
Vitamin D	√	√	√	
Vitamin E	√	√	√	√
Vitamin H (biotin or Vit B7)	√	√		√
Vitamin K	√	√	√	
Choline			√	
Folic Acid (B9)		√	√	√
Rutin		√		
Inositol		√	√	√
Calcium	√	√	√	√
Phosphorous	√	√	√	√
Iron	√	√	√	√
Copper	√	√		√
Potassium	√	√	√	
Magnesium	√	√	√	√
Manganese	√	√	√	
Silica		√		
Sulphur	√	√		
Sodium	√	√	√	
Iodine		√		√
Boron		√		
Zinc	√	√	√	√
Selenium		√	√	
	Moringa	Bee Pollen	Spirulina	Chlorella

Nutrient	Moringa	Bee Pollen	Spirulina	Chlorella
ENZYMES				
Disstase		√		
Phosphatase		√		
Amylase		√		
Cataiase		√		
Saccharase		√		
Diaphorase		√		
Pectase		√		
Cozymase		√		
Cytochrome		√		
AMINO ACIDS				
Alanine	√	√	√	√
Arginine	√	√	√	√
Aspartic Acid	√	√	√	
Cystine	√	√	√	√
Glutamic Acid	√	√	√	
Glycine	√	√	√	√
Histidine	√	√	√	√
Isoleucine	√	√	√	
Leucine	√	√	√	√
Lysine	√	√	√	√
Methionine	√	√	√	√
Phenylanaline	√	√	√	√
Proline	√	√	√	√
Threonine	√	√	√	
Tryptophan	√	√	√	√
Tyrosine	√	√	√	√
Valine	√	√	√	√
Chlorophyll	√		√	√
Protein	√	√	√	√
	Moringa	Bee Pollen	Spirulina	Chlorella

Spices

Cayenne

Good for the kidneys, lungs, spleen, pancreas, heart and stomach; provides carotene, vitamins A, B1, B2, B3, B5, B6, B9, and C; promotes weight loss; enhances immune system; fights Psoriasis; combats herpes, shingles, ulcers; stimulates appetite, aids digestion by stimulating gastric juices; reduces inflammation; increases blood flow to areas afflicted with rheumatism and arthritis; improves metabolism; relieves gas, colds, and stops bleeding from ulcers.

Cinnamon

Helps with constipation, coronary problems, diarrhea, digestive irritation indigestion, nausea and parasites. Use on fruits, porridge and smoothies.

Ginger

Boosts circulation; cures indigestion; combats inflammation; improves arthritis, fevers, headaches and toothaches; prevents motion sickness and menstrual cramps; reduces bloating, heartburn and flatulence; suppresses cancer cells. Sprinkle on fruits and porridge. Every meal should include some ginger.

Sea salt

Find a brand with no additives and no added iodine. Use for internal saltwater wash and cooking.

Supplements and Vitamins

Chlorophyll

Chlorophyll is the green pigment in all green plants and in cyanobacteria (blue-green algae, spirulina) responsible for the absorption of light that provides energy for photosynthesis (converting light into energy). If it's in every plant in Nature, then it must be essential! Chlorophyll fights carcinogens (cancercausing substances); deodorizes the body; reduces the effects of pollution in the system; is anti-oxidant and anti-inflammatory; helps chelate (bind with and remove) heavy metals like mercury; fights Candida Albicans and contains Vitamin K, C, folic acid, iron calcium, protein and magnesium. Real, living green plants are, of course, the best source of chlorophyll, but green powders and supplementation with liquid chlorophyll are acceptable substitutes.

Niacin

Niacin and other B complex vitamins are necessary for energy. They convert dietary proteins, fats, and carbohydrates into usable energy. Niacin synthesizes starch and stores in muscles and liver for future use as an energy source. It's found in barley, brown rice, some nuts and green vegetables. Its primary use in the Clean Cell Protocol is as an activating agent for the sauna "hot rinse" detox.

Green powder

Various manufacturers offer blends of various greens, vitamins, minerals, antioxidants, fiber, fruits, enzymes and probiotics in powder form. Green Vibrance™ is popular. I currently use Greens Pak™.

Vitamin C

Vitamin C is an antioxidant that strengthens the heart, builds immunity, clears bacteria, reduces cellular DNA damage, helps iron absorption, strengthens hair, delays signs of aging and more!

Vegan calcium

I keep a vegetarian source of calcium on hand for my teeth and bones. I use Vegan Cal-Mag by Veglife

Potassium

Potassium, along with sodium, chloride, calcium, and magnesium, is an electrolyte that is essential for life. It is found in nearly all foods (again, Nature's hint that this is important). I keep a potassium supplement to replenish what is lost during the hot rinse sauna.

Magnesium citrate

Another electrolyte to replace loss from sweating and sauna activities.

CHAPTER 9: Movement ▲

Movement Options

A certain amount of movement and sweating is necessary to keep the cells of the body clean. The prolonged sitting of modern work and leisure lifestyles leads to muscle degeneration, colon cancer, poor circulation, weak bones and even lowered brain function.

Run on the beach
When possible—if I'm on an island in the Pacific or southern China—I start my day with a 3 mile barefoot run on the beach. I get fresh air, grounding and sweating all at once.

Trampoline/rebounder
Trampolining has numerous benefits. By subjecting the entire body to gravitational forces, it has the unique effect of stimulating more of the body than even swimming! It increases the capacity for breathing. It circulates more oxygen to the tissues. It helps combat depression. It helps normalize blood pressure. It helps prevent cardiovascular disease. It increases the activity of the red bone marrow in the production of red blood cells. It aids lymphatic circulation, as well as blood flow in the veins of the circulatory system. It lowers elevated cholesterol and

triglyceride levels. It stimulates the metabolism thereby reducing the likelihood of obesity. It improves coordination throughout the body. It enhances digestion and elimination processes. It relieves fatigue and menstrual discomfort for women. It minimizes allergies, digestive disturbances, and abdominal problems. It tends to slow down aging.

Sources: www.busywomensfitness.com/rebounding.html
https://healingdaily.com/best-mini-trampolines/

Headstand

Lymph fluid (part of the lymphatic system) flowing through the body collects waste from the various organs and carries it to the bloodstream. Lymph is propelled through the body by physical activity, muscle contractions and gravity (that's why exercise in general, and rebounding are so beneficial). Inversion allows for the flow of lymph to hard-to-reach areas of the body by switching off the pull of gravity. Inversion reverses the blood flow and provides the brain with more oxygen which revitalizes. It helps the lymph move to the respiratory system; relieves back pain by reducing pressure on the nerves and discs in the spine; realigns the spine; improves joint health and builds "core" strength. In other words, it makes you younger!

Five Tibetan Rites of Rejuvenation

From a now public domain pamphlet by Peter Kelder called *The Eye of Revelation*, originally published in 1939, republished in 1999 under the title *Ancient Secret of the Fountain of Youth*, these 5 exercises "calibrate the body's seven energy centers (chakras) to spin harmoniously at the same speed in order to ensure the proper flow of vital life energy (prana) upward through the seven major endocrine glands (pineal, pituitary, thyroid, thymus, adrenals, pancreas, and testes [men] & ovaries [women])."

From a now public domain pamphlet by Peter Kelder called *The Eye of Revelation*, originally published in 1939, republished in 1999 under the title Ancient Secret of the Fountain of Youth, these 5 exercises "calibrate the body's seven energy centers (chakras) to spin harmoniously at the same speed in order to ensure the proper flow of vital life energy (prana) upward through the seven major endocrine glands (pineal, pituitary, thyroid, thymus, adrenals, pancreas, and testes [men] & ovaries [women])."

The book includes a secret sixth rite that is essential for maintaining youth. Check it out online!

CHAPTER 10: Expectations ▲

Expectations during the healing

Healing crisis vs. illness

Once you start aligning yourself with truth, encouraging flow and eating real healing foods, your body will start to react. There will be elimination, detoxification, rebalancing, regeneration and rejuvenation as you start to reactivate your body's healing code.

As we learned earlier, opposite conditions are just extreme ends of the same thing. Therefore, when your body starts to heal, you return back from illness along the same path that got you there (retracings). The road back from ill health towards good health will take you back through some of the same pain and discomfort you experienced on the original journey.

In the case of detoxification, for instance, many of the toxins that are now lodged in your tissues will be loosened and find their way back into your bloodstream on their way to your kidneys and ultimately out of your system. That will result in certain symptoms of "illness" returning as you heal. In other words, you may feel worse while you're getting better. This is what we call a healing crisis.

Those crises may include nausea, vomiting headaches, sleepiness, frequent bowel movements or urination, rumbling in the stomach, sweating and occasional pains in parts of the body being healed.

Remember, Nature's road is a slow single lane. You are accomplishing a transition from disease to health. This transitional period cannot be rushed. Most real cure cannot happen overnight. Part of the new paradigm involves respecting the intelligence of gradual cure at Nature's pace. It takes a certain degree of discipline to maintain a new transitional lifestyle while Nature does its thing.

Yes, reversing aging is a process. Enter into this process with the understanding that you're taking your body backwards along a path towards good health. There will be days you feel better and days you feel worse. The key is to resolve to stick it out. Don't worry about the bad days. All you're doing is putting fruits and vegetables into your body. There's essentially nothing you're doing that's harmful. So any discomfort you feel is likely what's called a "die-off" reaction (i.e., healing crisis), or your body adjusting itself to the new diet. The experience itself will teach you much about health, your body, as well as the true nature of illness and healing.

Expectations for the sequence of rejuvenation

Things are happening inside your body of which you may be unaware. These are things happening on subtle levels, on tissue levels, on inner organ levels that are not having visible manifestations. Your body knows. When you start a healing and rejuvenation protocol, your body will send the nutrients or facilitate the cleansing of particular systems and organs that need to be healed before other systems can be healed. Before healing your skin condition, for example, your body may need to heal your liver since the liver is a major organ of detoxification. Trust that your body's innate intelligence is at work to reverse the deterioration in the appropriate sequence. This is why discipline, patience and consistency are essential for any true healing.

The instantaneous, overnight, magic pill type of healing that we've been led to expect from healing treatments is really just the suppression of symptoms. It is not real healing. Real healing, just like the real deterioration that took years of bad living to develop, may also take some time to reverse.

The good news, however, is that while it does take some time, it often does not take as many years to heal as it did to fall ill. I've heard some practitioners say it takes 1 month of healing for every 1 year of deterioration. I've heard others say it takes 2 weeks for every 1 year. It doesn't really matter who's correct. The point is, you must respect the natural sequence and trust your body's intelligence.

Expectations as a result of the healing

If the results of your experiment resemble mine and my friends', you might experience:

Increased sexual energy

Now, I don't want to appear egotistical. I don't want it to seem as if I'm fishing or auditioning for girlfriends, but I can tell you from my own experience that, as a result of my clean cell lifestyle:

My erections are stronger now than when I was in college. I can perform for an average of three hours or more, and since I choose not to ejaculate during sex (another component of my "Fit to Breed" practices), I maintain a high level of arousal that I sublimate into creative endeavors like writing.

Benefits people notice

"I don't want to be inappropriate," he began, "but if you don't mind me saying so, you have an aura of peace that I don't see too often in people."

That's what my doorman, Irving, said to me recently. We had seen each other only briefly amid quick hellos and goodbyes as I made my way hastily in and out on various errands. Today, however, he felt compelled to stop me to chat for a bit.

Although I often don't recall the compliments people give me, this one stood out. It put a smile on my face, and a little extra pep and peace in my step all that day, and even now when I think about it. I thanked him greatly for it at the time.

"An aura of peace." That has to be the greatest compliment I've received recently. It stands as validation of the discipline, the consistency and the effort I've put in throughout these years to live the lifestyle. It says to me that not only are the effects of my beliefs and choices evident to me in how I feel physically, but they are visible to others in qualitative ways that transcend mere physical appearance.

The deterioration we associate with this thing called aging is a function of being out of alignment with truth mentally, physically and spiritually. Clean cell living is based on truth. The search for those truths puts you on a path of discovery. The discovery of those truths puts you on a path of awakening. The adoption of those truths frees you from deception, puts you in control of your health, and sets your mind, body and spirit in alignment with universal truth.

If my doorman Irving's observation of my aura is to be believed, one cannot help but exude an aura of peace when one is in alignment with truth.

It is my greatest wish that *you* experience the same alignment, get compliments, live long and prosper!

Beauty that stands out
Here's an actual email from a client and friend:

"I was walking to the train station on my way to the gym. A guy who was entering the train kept watching me. I continued on my way and shortly after found him staring my way while on the platform.

After the gym, I headed to get lunch. I was looking at the outside menu and wondering if I had the time wrong as it was past noon and they were supposed to be open by then. A man behind me asked if I knew when they opened. After answering him we stood waiting for a minute when he blurted out "If you don't mind my saying so, you look so young."

I saw you from behind and you turned around and I thought you looked 18!

After lunch, I went to get my son from school. As I crossed the street by the school, a guy coming towards me said, "You look beautiful, mami." Later, while walking to the grocery store, a guy stopped and said, "My gosh you are simply beautiful, girl!" When I thanked him, he replied, "No, thank you!" On my walk back from the store a guy passing me threw me a kiss.

My question to you is: What's IN this stuff I'm taking?????!"

"Yes, but what about my gray hair???"

Many people start to worry about aging once they

notice some gray hairs. Even though there can be many causes of gray hair, for the most part, I've found the condition—while undeniably exacerbated by stress—is really a mineral deficiency. I've had friends/clients notice a decrease in gray hair both on the head and in the pubic area, once they've been on the Clean Cell protocol. Everything is reversible!

That's just my own few experiences. There are tens of thousands more online and in the archives and case histories of alternative healers worldwide.

Expectations from the masses

Depending on your social circles, you should also expect a certain amount of resistance from friends, family, strangers and even health care providers:

"Why don't you just live a normal life without going to all these extremes? What are you a germophobe?"
This is not about being germophobic. We live in a world in which what's normal is unnatural. In other words, what you refer to as a "normal" life has already forced you and the cells of your body to the extremes of an unnatural existence. It is unnatural to breathe exhaust fumes every day, eat chemicals and call it fine dining, subsist entirely on non-living food, live in unnatural light, etc. Clean cell living is simply taking action in response to the corrosive, deteriorating

effects of what we now consider normal living, through the deliberate exercise of strategies to return your body and its environment to a cleaner, more natural state.

"Everything in moderation, I always say!"

"Moderation" is a strategy often advocated by those without the discipline to curb their appetites, or those with a food product to sell. It allows drunkards, addicts and the weak-willed to feel better about their behavior because any level of indulgence in an addictive vice can be passed off as moderation. You, however, cannot afford to be moderate in your experiment in immortality. As we said earlier:

Extremism in defense of health is not a vice. Moderation in pursuit of immortality is no virtue.

5 Reasons we won't start with a fast

Even though an extended water fast is one of the best ways to "re-boot" your body's digestive and elimination systems, there are a few reasons why we won't start with a long one right away

1. We DON'T want your introduction to clean cell living to feel like it's all about deprivation.

2. We DO want to immediately stop putting garbage into your body and replace your intake with real food.

3. We DO want to develop good eating habits before the fast, so they can be easily resumed after.

4. It's likely your absorption and elimination are operating at sub-par levels. So as much as possible, even with that limitation, we are going to provide the body with certain nutrients to improve absorption and elimination before fasting.

5. It's possible you have parasites, which would lower your energy level while on a fast. Therefore, in addition to the replacement diet, we're going to do a parasite cleanse first and the flow of bulk through the system (eating) will help.

Do something, anything, immediately!

Things you can do even while reading this book:

☐ *Throw stuff away*

Go to your kitchen right now and throw away white sugar, white flour, table salt, anything with MSG, corn syrup or fructose, canned goods, dairy products and coffee (if it's plain, organic coffee, save it and use for enemas). Yes, throw it away! If you really believe it is poison, you can't, in good conscience, give it to someone else, now can you?

☐ *Squat right*

Set up a bucket, box, upside-down basin or purchase a squatty-potty-type product to elevate your knees for better evacuation.

☐ *Begin a 24-hour fast*

Commit to doing nothing but drink water for a full 24 hours until this precise time tomorrow.

☐ *Go shopping*

Go shopping at a health food store and/or produce market (see substitution/shopping list and acid/alkaline chart) and include substitutions for items you regularly use or enjoy (cereal, cheese, sweeteners, etc.)

Clean Cell SUBSTITION Shopping List

AVOID: Milk, butter, eggs, cheese, chicken, all meats processed sugar and salt, all foods with artificial flavor, preservatives & color of any kind, alcohol cigarettes, sodas, fried foods, hybrid rice and wheat products, processed white flour, decaffeinated coffee, all hybrid and genetically modified foods

ITEMS TO AVOID	REPLACE WITH
white sugar	maple syrup, honey, agave
white rice	brown rice, millet, quinoa
white flour	flour from rice, almond, lentil
animal milk	soy, almond or rice milk
soda, alcohol, canned juices,	Fresh juices, water, coconut water, herbal teas
meat	curried eggplant, mushrooms, lentil, stewed peas, soy-based faux meat products
animal-based cheese	soy or rice cheese
coffee, tea	herb teas
butter, margarine	olive oil, palm oil
table salt	sea salt, rock salt, celtic salt
grain vinegar	apple cider vinegar, coconut vinegar
canned products	fresh, living foods
canola cooking oil	coconut oil

Clean Cell Shopping List

FRUIT/VEGGIES
Choice of fruits
squash
avocado
beets
string beans
eggplants
okra
red/green pepper
Brussels sprouts
asparagus
collard greens
turnip greens
radish
cabbage
purslane
yellow dock
sheppards purse
dandelion greens
dasheen greens
green papaya

Power Salad
spinach
watercress
parsley
celery
cucumber

OILS
flax seed oil
virgin coconut oil
pumpkin seed oil
virgin olive oil

SEAWEED
spirulina powder
dulse flakes
kelp powder
Irish moss

HERBS/Bitters
Echinacea
wood root tonic
sea salt
cayenne pepper

MEAT SUBS
tofu, mushrooms
seitan
bean curd
mock meats

SWEETENERS
honey, agave
maple syrup
stevia

SUPPLEMENTS
bee pollen
royal jelly
tissue salts
liq multi-vitamin
B-12 drops
mineral drops
lecithin
nutritional yeast
app cider vinegar
molasses
Acidophilus

GRAINS
quinoa
millet
brown rice
barley

BATH
soap
tea tree oil
loofah brush

MISCELLANY
raw snacks
dried fruit
nuts

Shopping Tip

As a clean cell shopper, it's important to know that all brands are not created equal. Not all labels are truthful. Not all ingredient labels reveal what's actually in a product. One rule of thumb I'll share with you is that any products from corporate conglomerates that have recently jumped on the health food bandwagon are probably not to be trusted.

You see, large, publicly traded corporations and concerns have a mandate to increase profits to benefit their shareholders. Their primary concern, therefore, is to reduce costs by finding the cheapest labor and products, and thus increase profits. That means mass produced, factory grown, industrially-farmed products sometimes contain genetically-modified ingredients.

Though things are changing, it's generally a safe bet to assume that the products you need in order to implement the Clean Cell lifestyle won't be found in your neighborhood supermarket or bodega. You'll likely have to change where you shop.

Smaller, sometimes individually or family-owned businesses and brands that started out in the health field are usually a better choice. They are usually found in smaller health food stores. Their products often have to be ordered directly. You can find these companies by doing a bit of research online. Their names will become more familiar over time.

A friend of mine once remarked:

"Walt, when I go to the supermarket and pick up organic fruits, how do I even know for sure that it's organic? I'd hate to be fooled into paying more for stuff that's not really organic! I'd rather just keep buying the regular stuff rather than be duped."

That's a valid concern. Consider this, however:

The concept of "organic" produce is not a figment of someone's imagination. It is real. There IS such a thing as "organic" produce. To that we can all agree.

Next, industry standards have been developed which dictate the criteria growers must meet before they are allowed to label and sell their items as "organic." The fact is, the majority of people who are labeling their products as such are not attempting to trick you. We have to trust to some degree that people are watching—that there is someone making sure the growers are adhering to those standards. Yes, there is definitely a bit of trust and faith involved.

Further, you can often see and taste the difference between conventionally-grown and organic. Organic produce will often look less "shiny-perfect" than the GMO/industrially grown stuff.

Yes, there can be deception. There can be mislabeling anywhere along the process, but those who violate the standards know there will be consequences. At the end of the day, you just have to trust that the system works (that industry standards are being enforced, that agencies are doing their jobs, that honest people exist, that labeling guidelines are followed), that people are watching for and investigating scams, and take your chances.

Not wanting to be "duped" is not a sufficient reason to ignore your health. You can't let your pride prevent you from living a potentially life-saving lifestyle.

Do this in phase I

☐ *Start taking the green juice cocktails*
    Take either with apple juice or with a juice from your juicer. Take chlorella, spirulina and/or barley grass to replenish vitamins and minerals. This is a necessary step so that your body will be strong enough for the cleanses, the fasting and the sauna detox.

☐ *Perform a coffee enema*
    One coffee enema can change your life! Perform one early on to start the purging process.

☐ *Schedule a colonic*
    A colonic is a procedure best done by a qualified practitioner. I can tell you from my own experience

that no matter how clean you may believe your system to be, it can benefit from a colonic. My first colonic experience was seven days of a daily colonic, supplemented with green juice and clay and psyllium throughout the day.

At the time, I had already been vegan for about ten years and felt I only needed a single day's colonic evacuation. I reluctantly agreed to the seven-day program at the insistence of my hygienist. On the fourth day, the worms came out! I'll spare you the photos! Guess she knew what she was doing, after all! Sure, there are other ways to get at those pesky worms that may be lodged deep in your colon, but I swear by colonics because of my own positive experience!

☐ *Start taking chlorophyll and oxygen*
Take oxygen in the form of food grade hydrogen peroxide along with 100mg liquid chlorophyll.

☐ *Do the blood work*
A single drop of blood from a pinprick, analyzed under a microscope and explained by an experienced naturopath can show you parasites (if any), blood cells, as well as the effects of poor diet and dehydration on the clustering and movement of your cells. This step is not critical, but would be a good "before" snapshot to compare later after you've been on the protocol.

☐ *Address parasites if necessary*

If the blood work or symptoms indicate you have parasites, then you need to address them immediately. Take oil of oregano, grapefruit seed extract, wormwood, a parasite cleanse product, or see my own protocol in *"16-inch Worms in My Toilet...with photos"* at www.agelessadept.com/resources (also posted at curezone.org)

Do this during phase II

☐ *Experience your first water fast*
Full instructions: www.fastandgrowyoung.com

☐ *Do your first detox "hot rinse" sauna*
Full instructions: see: www.agelessadept.com/resources

☐ *Perform a system cleanse (colon, kidney, liver)*
Details: www.huldaclark.net

☐ *Start moving*

Movement of the body is vital to maintaining youth. Exercise! Rebounding is a great method to get the lymph moving through your system.

Now that you know the therapies in the Clean Cell Protocol, and have moved past the initial transition and focus phases, your next step is to incorporate them into your daily life. It's easier than you think.

A Suggested Morning Routine

• Do oil pulling during your morning routine
• Rinse mouth with GSE-water
• Drink lemon water, GSE-water or something alkalizing
• Evacuate in a squatting position as necessary
• Place a few drops of Universal Remedy* under tongue
• Shower with water from your water filter
• If you're not fasting, eat a fruit breakfast

See section on Urine Therapy

A Suggested Exercise Routine

• Jump for 5-10 minutes on a rebounder
• Invert/headstand for 5 minutes (with care)
• Perform the 6 Rites
• Run, jog, speed-walk, cycle

My list of "secrets"

Someone asked me to make a list of the things I did, and the things I do (or don't do) that account for my youthfulness and strength. Here's that actual list: *passion-centered lifestyle, sunshine, water, earth, air, time, issue-specific herbs and supplements, coffee / chlorophyll / h202 enemas, sauna "hot rinse" detox, wash hair with spring water, no soap on face, one meal per day; no food after 4pm, green juice, running in the sun, sunbathing, fasting, veganism, coconut water and fruit juice, raw food, spirulina, cook with coconut oil only, no car, no air con, zapper, diatomaceous earth, no chemicals on skin, no shaving cream, no antiperspirant, passion-centered life, personal growth, MMS, DMSO, GSE, MSM, ejaculate once per month, headstand/inversion.*

According to my paradigm, the only two causes of illness are insufficient nutrition and/or inadequate waste removal. Therefore, any health issue I've ever needed to address (for me and my friends)--gray hairs, congestion, body odor, low energy, low libido, pain, parasites, constipation, weakening eyesight--has been addressed with something on the list. Some are an ongoing lifestyle, others are issue-related, others for prevention. This chart, based on my own experiences, suggests how often they may be practiced.

Issue-specific	Every day	Once-twice/wee	Once-twice/month
MMS DMSO Oil of oregano Herbs Fast	One main meal 12-3pm (Vitalized meal) GSE in food MSM in food Sprg water shampoo Green juice Coconut water Fresh juice/nectar Spirulina Cook w/coconut oil Diatomaceous earth Rebounder	Sunbath Run on beach Chlorophyll enema H2O2 enema Headstand /invert	Coffee enema Hot rinse sauna Zapper session Ejaculation

*No antiperspirant, shaving cream, lotions, pesticides, flavorings, drugs.
*No sugar, coffee, sodas, alcohol

CHAPTER 12: A Few Recipes ▲

Activate your body's healing code with tasty, natural meals that provide nutrients & help remove waste

Vitalize your food

Congratulations! Now that you accept that food isn't just about taste, your food can now be vitalized, energized and empowered! Remember we learned that

Vitality = Potential Power minus Obstruction

That potential power is a function of the nutrition in the food you eat (as well as your body's ability to digest and assimilate it). To ensure your meals provide you with the optimum amount of vitality, you'll need to ask different questions as you prepare them:

How can I make this meal better? How can I make this meal more alkaline, more nutritious and/or more cleansing? Can I add something raw and living to this meal? Here are examples of how to do that:

At breakfast, mix a teaspoon of calcium powder into your oatmeal. Stir silica-rich diatomaceous earth into your porridge. Sprinkle nutritionally-complete bee pollen onto your gluten-free waffles after you pour on the mineral-rich Grade B maple syrup.

While preparing your main meal, put a few germ-killing, alkalizing drops of grapefruit seed extract

(GSE) in with your maple syrup-sweetened lemonade. Sprinkle an ounce of high-fatty acid, fiber-rich chia seeds onto your salad or mixed into your brown rice. Add cleansing apple cider vinegar to your salad. Throw a spoonful of nutrient-loaded, chlorophyll-rich spirulina powder onto your stir-fry. Empower your barley or millet with omega-rich pumpkin seed oil. Make any meal a natural antibiotic with pressed garlic cloves. Put some bee pollen and maca powder into your smoothies. Make every meal more warming and easy to assimilate with some cayenne pepper and ginger! Vitalize your food!

A word about the recipes

You are now eating not just for taste, but for clean cells. Each ingredient in these recipes serves a purpose: to provide nutrients or cleansing. Omit the sprouts and you won't get living enzymes. You can't substitute Splenda® for maple syrup just because that's what you have in your cupboard. They are not the same simply because they both taste sweet. One is a natural food, the other is a poison.

Add a little more/less of any ingredient according to your preference, but keep the ingredient in place.

BREAKFASTS

Raw Reversal Porridge
Vitality quotient: high

- ½ cup grated dry coconut
- 1 grated sweet potato
- 1 banana
- ¼ cup trail mix*
- cinnamon

- Vitalize with bee pollen, flax seeds, pumpkin seeds

*avoid dried fruit with added sugar and sulfites

Forever Fruit Bowl
Vitality quotient: medium

- cubed papaya or apples or pears
- sliced banana
- Gluten-free waffles
- Organic maple syrup
- Vitalize with bee pollen, blackstrap molasses

Perpetual Purple Porridge (cooked)
Vitality quotient: basic

- rice flour (grind your own brown rice)
- grated green banana* & grated purple sweet potato*
- oatmeal
- Vitalize with calcium, diatomaceous earth, psyllium husk right before eating; do not cook these.

Bring water to boil, add each ingredient in order listed at 2-3 minute intervals.

Vitality notes:
*purple sweet potato: Okinawan longevity staple
*banana: potassium

MAIN MEAL

"Raw Power Slaw"
Vitality Quotient:high

Ingredients:
- ½ med Napa cabbage
- ½ cup sprouted lentils
- ¼ cup malunggay leaves
- 1 avocado
- 2 pressed garlic cloves
- 2 tbs apple cider vinegar
- dash of sea salt
- dash of cayenne pepper
- one chopped scallion
- 2 tsp spirulina powder

Directions:
- Shred/chop cabbage; add avocado, crush into slaw-like mixture with cabbage; finely chop malunggay and add with all other ingredients and mix
- optional to taste: grated ginger, chia seeds, finely diced onions, grated carrots, celery, sea weed
- Vitalize even more with apple cider vinegar, or pumpkin seed oil or nutritional yeast

Serving suggestion: Eat with natural chips
Vitality notes:
- Sprouts: a raw, living, enzyme-rich food
- Malunggay: multi vitamins and minerals
- Apple cider vinegar: bodily, intestinal cleansing
- Garlic: a natural antibacterial
- Spirulina, mineral/protein/chlorophyll-rich algae
- Cayenne: improves circulation, aids digestion

<u>Jamaican Rice & Peas</u>
Vitality Quotient: basic

Ingredients:
- 2½ -3 cups water
- 1 cup brown rice
- 1 cup kidney beans
- 1 cup grated dry coconut
- dash of sea salt
- 1 scallion stalk chopped

Directions:
- Soak kidney beans overnight
- Soak grated coconut in water, then squeeze out water through strainer or cloth.
- Combine all ingredients in pot or pressure cooker
- Bring water to boil for 5 minutes
- Medium-low for 30-40 min (pressure cook: 15 min).
- Vitalize with spirulina, pumpkin seed oil

<u>"Longevity Soup" (Congee)</u>
Vitality Quotient: high

Ingredients:
brown rice, teff, food herbs, millet, black beans (optional), distilled/filtered water, crock pot.

Directions:
Pour ¼ cup of each grain (millet, rice, teff) into the pot. Add beans. Fill to brim with water, cover and cook on low overnight. Serve hot. Pour over greens. Vitalize with dulse, spirulina, other herbs

Vitality notes:
- Dissolves fat, strengthens kidneys, reverses aging. Buddha refers to congee as "the food of longevity."

SECRETS FROM MY VITALITY VAULT

<u>"Comeback Cocktail"</u>
An original concoction that keeps me going strong!
Vitality Quotient: off the chart!

Ingredients:
- 12-16oz coconut water or apple juice
- 1-2 oz apl cider vinegar
- 1 tbsp maca
- 1 tbsp chlorophyll (100mg)
- 1 tbsp black seed oil
- 1 pack greens powder
- 1 pack electrolyte powder
- 3-5 drops GSE
- 1oz trace minerals*
- 1oz DMSO

Directions:
Combine all ingredients, close jar, and shake! Open carefully. The electro-mix can cause a pressure buildup! The amounts are flexible. Use more or less of each as you choose. May have a cleansing effect the first time.
*Some trace minerals taste salty. Sun Warrior Liquid Light has a pleasant taste that won't overpower.

<u>"Superhero Salad"</u>
Vitality Quotient: high

A staple you can have at every meal. The ingredients can change based on seasonal availability or taste: alfalfa, spinach, water cress, kale, radish, apple cider vinegar, lemon, liquid amino, sprinkle with dulse flakes, kelp, spirulina, lecithin, nutritional yeast.

A Clean Cell from Head to Toe
Habits, nutrients & cleanses for organs and systems

Hair: wash with spring water, shower filter; no sodium lauryl sulfate (SLS) in shampoos; soaps; take mineral supplement

Lungs: no air condition;deep breathing; no smoking; get air purifier; no air fresheners

Joints: MSM, movement, exercise

Skin: No shaving cream or chemicals; expose to sunlight; virgin coconut oil; hot rinse sauna; put nothing on the body you can't put in the body; brush massage

Liver: coffee enema

Heart: cayenne; no fried food; alkalizing foods; no hydrogenated oils; vegan diet

Reproductive system: no birth control (IUDs, pills, sponges); no chemicals to induce erections; no fluorescent lights

Blood: Echinacea, dandelion and other blood cleansers

Digestion: caloric restriction, yearly fast; raw living food, fiber, colonics, fasts; parasite cleanse; take digestive enzymes

Lymph nodes:
rebounder; deep tissue/Swedish massage; inversion
Brain:
remove mercury fillings from teeth No fluoroscent lighting

A Clean Cell
Sunlight, water, earth, air and time

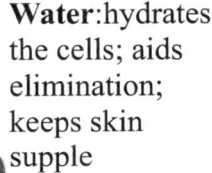

Sunlight: encourages Vit D production; kills germs on skin; improves mood. Do not use sunblock

Water:hydrates the cells; aids elimination; keeps skin supple

Earth: grounds body; cleanses colon in the form of clay;

Air: oxygenates the cells of the body;

Time: Allows healing at nature's pace;

LAUNCH CEREMONY:
The Final Motivational Speech ▲

"[Carrel] maintained the living culture for well over 20 years...proving that living cells could be kept alive indefinitely by simply controlling the nutrients and removing the waste in the surrounding solution.

Proper nutrition and removal of waste. This is the simple formula for longevity for which no practical lifestyle guide has ever existed." **--Chapter 1**

So there you have it: the Clean Cell Living Protocol--you now have a practical lifestyle guide for conducting your very own experiment in longevity (and perhaps bodily immortality)--a practical way to duplicate Carrel's experiment of nutrient and waste removal. In its simplest terms, it shows you how to:
• Cleanse the body of toxic accumulations
• Substitute and prepare nutrient-rich, real food
• Adopt a set of habits to live pristinely (cleanly), and activate the body's foolproof healing code for repair, reversal & rejuvenation

Entire books, libraries, careers and communities have been written, compiled, launched and coalesced around each of these practices and products. Far from being an exhaustive treatise, therefore, this book is an introduction to give you enough information to assess each one's value to your body and to inform additional research and investigation for your life experiment.

Many of these treatments are effective, easy to use, and cheap. Consequently, they pose a threat to the profits of established treatments. Don't be surprised, therefore, if you find articles online that speak of dangers, doubt, uncertainty, lack of evidence or the need for more scientific research. I and many others have used them and have had no harmful side effects.

In order to conduct *your* experiment, you need to start with some basic truths. These truths are not up for debate. This is not an exercise in free speech and freedom of choice. This is not one man's opinion he's "entitled to." Sure, you have the freedom to choose to eat a raw or a cooked carrot, but make no mistake, the consequences of each of those choices are not equal.

A raw carrot is better for your body. Period.

The only people who engage in debate about these truths are (a) people who lack the courage and discipline to change their habits, and (b) people who and entities that stand to gain financially from maintaining the status quo.

When it comes to these truths, your agreement is irrelevant. Your opinion is immaterial. What you like (or don't like) really doesn't matter.

For instance, MSM is in most raw foods, but is

destroyed in the cooking process. What that means is, if you were eating more raw food, you would automatically be healthier since you'd be receiving higher amounts of MSM. So, whether you "like" raw foods or not does not change the fact that the body is designed to function optimally with it.

Whether you choose to engage in a vegetarian lifestyle or not doesn't change the fact that your body was designed to thrive on fruits and vegetables.

Whether you like sunbathing or not does not change the fact the body was designed to function optimally with exposure to the sun.

No other animal in nature drinks the milk of another species. This is aberrant behavior, and it comes with consequences.

The soil in which your food is grown is depleted of vital nutrients. Whether you eat organic food or not doesn't change the fact that your body requires such nutrients in order for function optimally.

"...but I don't like broccoli!"

You've been led to believe that your diet is a matter of choosing what you like and avoiding what you don't like. You've been led to believe you can eat canned vegetables, fast food, processed substances, and that you'll be okay.

You've been misled.

I suggest you not waste the valuable moments of your life arguing on behalf of maintaining a lifestyle and lie-style that is provably false and destructive to your body. I suggest you not argue "everything in moderation" as a way to justify and rationalize your bad habits. I suggest you not allow advertising, pharmaceutical companies, dairy councils and meat lobbies to convince you that milk does a body good or that meat is real food for real people.

In other words, eating raw food, eliminating milk and dairy products, stopping the ingestion of faux foods and all the suggestions in the Clean Cell Protocol are not just interesting ideas for you to ponder and choose from like a buffet. For each idea you adopt, you improve your health. For each idea you disregard, your health suffers.

If you're eating raw food, but still drinking the milk of cows, you can be healthy only to a limited degree. Yes, you can be healthier, but there will be a limit to the full expression of your body's healing and rejuvenation code.

Sure sounds like fanaticism or extremism, doesn't it? Well, I suppose it is. However, neither you nor I makes the rules. Nature does. I don't make the consequences. Nature does. Nature says that people who eat processed food for all their lives develop clogged arteries and suffer heart attacks. That's not my opinion or my rule. That's a provable reality.

Nature is what it is. The rates of cancer, heart disease, etc., are nothing more than humans suffering the consequences of violating Nature's laws in many ways. There is no getting around this. You cannot violate the law and escape the consequences.

The Clean Cell Protocol offers you a set of practices that, as regularly-practiced habits, can put you in alignment with Nature's laws as much as practical in modern society. Some people will be more successful than others. Some people will have the required courage and discipline. Some people will have the support of family and environment.

If you do not have the courage or discipline; if you do not have the support of family and environment; if your current lifestyle, job or home situation, relationship, neighborhood and belief system are not conducive to adopting the protocol, there is nothing I can offer as a "work around." This is as close to a magic pill as it gets.

There is no substitute that works as well as real food in the body. There is no substitute that works as well as real sunshine on the skin. There is no reasonable facsimile that works as well as fresh, clean air in the lungs. This protocol is the best there is, and whether you "like" broccoli or not doesn't change these facts. I leave you now, therefore, with some motivation for your journey in the form of a promise:

The Clean Cell Promise

"If you can find the courage and discipline to eat only what exists in Nature, avoid unnatural substances and environments, bask daily in sunshine, maintain direct contact with the earth, breathe clean air, purge the colon, cleanse the system, fast when dis-eased, and live passionately and on purpose from a belief system of universal perfection... you can keep the cells of the body clean, prevent illness, reverse aging, rejuvenate the body, achieve perfect health and long life and become your own fountain of youth!"

- "A clean cell never dies!"

Your Experiment Resource List ▲

| = products I've not personally tried...yet!

☐ Vitaminlife.com

☐ HealQuick.com *(formerly www.thecleaner.com*

☐ Discovermms.com *(MMS)*

☐ DrClark.com *(Zappers, organ cleanses)*

☐ The Ultimate Zapper http://zap.intergate.ca *(see archive.org)*

☐ Sota.com *(colloidal silver maker, water ozonator)*

☐ CrystalQuest.com *(shower water filter)*

☐ Cellcore.com *(Mimosa Pudica & Klinghardt protocol)*

☐ Statmx.com *(organic coffee; Gerson Therapy items)*

☐ Sawilsons.com *(recommended by enema therapy experts)*

☐ Ariseandshine.com *(Dr Anderson's colon kits)*

☐ ProHealthsolutions.com (cleanses, probiotics, enzymes)

☐ Globalhealthtrax.com (Global Health Trax probiotics)

☐ BIONATAL.CO (Black Seed oil; use coupon code AGELESS)

Books for more information

☐ *Prescription for Nutritional Healing* by Phyllis & James Balch; THE resource of natural remedies (vitamins, herbs, supplements) for common ailments.

☐ *Arnold Ehret's Mucusless Diet & Healing System* by A. Ehret; Ehret explores the single underlying cause of all disease and explains it in lay language.

☐ *Rational Fasting* by Arnold Ehret; A sequel.

☐ *The Master Cleanser* by Stanley Burroughs; Instructions for the "lemonade fast."

☐ *Diet For a New America* by John Robbins; the son of the founder of Baskin & Robbins Ice Cream exposes the horrendous and unsanitary conditions underlying the entire dairy and meat industries.

☐ *Back to Eden* by Jethro Kloss; An amazing resource of herbs and natural remedies.

☐ *Why Do Vegetarians Eat Like That?* by David Gabbe; No longer in print, but still available online,

☐ *Healing the Gerson Way* by Charlotte Gerson

☐ *Natural Cures They Don't Want You to Know* by Kevin Trudeau; An amazing expose, resource, guidebook!

☐ *Mad Cowboy* by Howard F. Lyman, Glen Merzer

☐ *Sugar Blues* by William Dufty

☐ *The Body Ecology Diet* by Donna Gates

☐ *Foods that Heal* by Bernard Jensen

☐ *How to Eat to Live* by Elijah Muhammad

☐ *Cleanse & Purify Thyself* by Richard Anderson

☐ *Blue Zones: 9 Lessons for Living Longer from the People who've lived the Longest* by Dan Buettner

Books for improved vitality/virility

☐ *Ancient Secret of the Fountain of Youth* by Peter Kelder; Originally published as T*he Eye of Revelation.*

☐ *The Tao of Sexology* by Dr. Stephen T. Chang

Books for universal truth

☐ *The Kybalion* (in the public domain)

Videos to change the world (or, at least, <u>your</u> life!)

☐ *The Gerson Miracle-* cure for cancer and all disease

☐ *The Beautiful Truth* - cancer cure

☐ *Seeds of Death* and other award-winning documentaries www.youtube.com/user/GaryNullTV

Websites for health information

- Whfoods.com; world's Healthiest Foods
- GaryNull.com; website of Gary Null
- Curezone.org/forums
- Healyourselfathome.com
- WellnessMama.com
- Educate-yourself.org
- Shirleys-wellness-cafe.com
- Livestrong.com
- EarthClinic.com
- Gerson.org; Charlotte Gerson's Gerson Therapy

~~~

Immortality in 17 syllables ▲
Eat real food only
Remove waste regularly
*Rinse and repeat--***Ageless Haiku**

Who is the Ageless Adept? ▲

"Perfect health, long life and eternal youth are not the random, genetic blessings of a chaotic or capricious universe, but natural birthrights that can be accessed through the mindful acceptance of simple truths, activated by the disciplined practice of proven protocols, and sustained by advancement along a known path. This is that path."

My name is Walt F.J. Goodridge, author and publisher of the *Ageless Adept*™ series of books. Years ago, before I became vegan, a friend asked a question over lunch I couldn't answer. He asked, *"Do you know what's in the food you're eating?"* I did not, and it bothered me that I didn't, and so--with health, longevity and vitality as my goals--I dedicated my life to a search for answers and ultimately to *"share what I know, so that others may grow."*

My childhood in the Caribbean gave me an understanding of and reverence for our natural world of sunshine, water, earth, air and time. As an adult, I discovered that what passes as *normal* health and healing in the western paradigm is shockingly *unnatural*! It never made sense to me that we should need to turn to men in lab coats with pills in search of wellness. It makes more sense that Nature would have the answers built in; our bodies would have an innate healing code; our "operations manual" would be simple and foolproof.

Through my experiments, testimonials from like mind,s and corroboration of researchers from this and previous eras, I've realized that the symptoms we accept as "normal" aging are the body's reactions to unnatural habits of ingesting pharmaceuticals, fake food with non-food ingredients, pesticides, hormones, steroids and antibiotics, as well as other environmental factors. Some habits may be hard to break, but are ultimately under our control. And, if the *causes* are controllable, then the *effects* are not inevitable and may even be reversible! That's what I'm here to prove!

I've distilled the results of my experiments into my Ageless Adept™ philosophy and protocols--information I hope will empower you to become your own authority in matters of health, and make better survival decisions when choosing from among the products and practices you'll encounter on your own path of perfect health, long life and the fountain of youth! So, who is the Ageless Adept? With the right choices, it will be you!

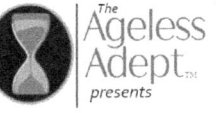
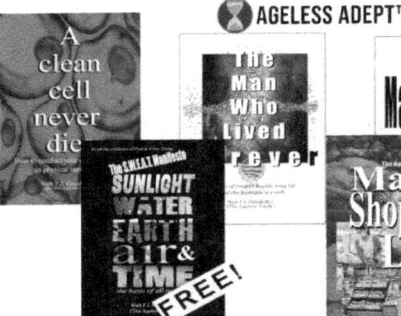
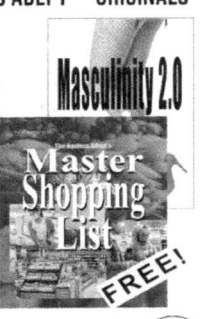
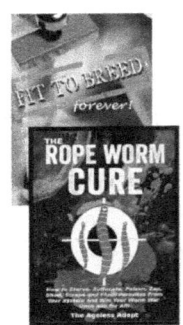
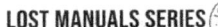
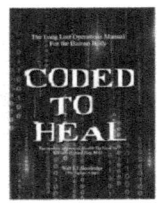
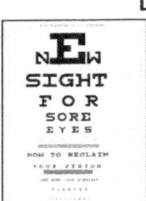
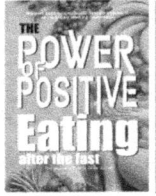
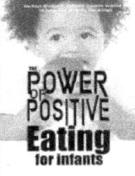
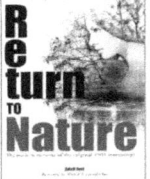
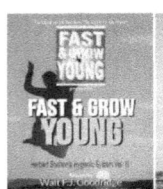
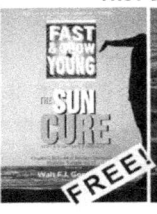
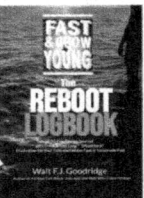
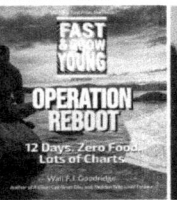
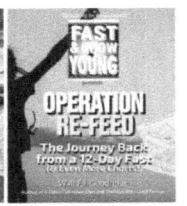

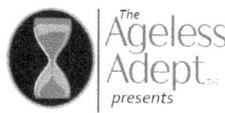

Ageless Adept Resources ▲

Infographics, posters and charts available at
www.agelessadept.com/downloads

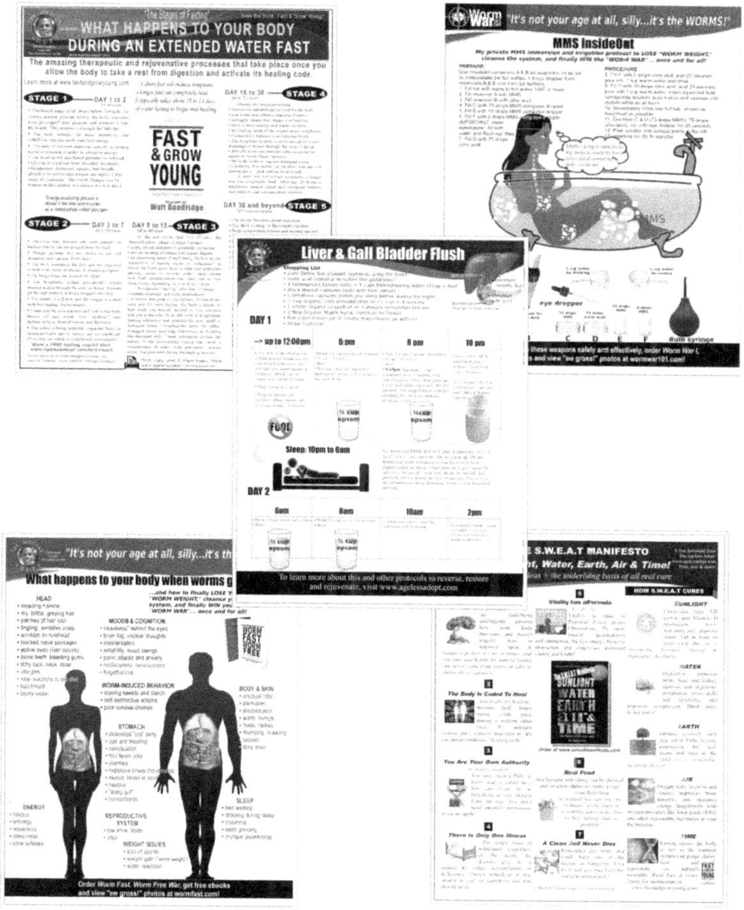

Book summaries, infographics, posters, charts with information and instructions for fasting, detoxing, parasite elimination and ageless living are available at www.agelessadept.com/downloads

Watch, Read, Wear & Learn ▲

Youtube™ Channels

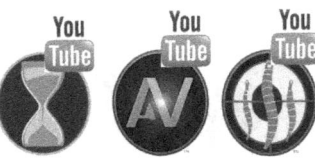

@agelessadept
@askavegan
@ropewormcure

Blogs

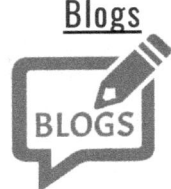

agelessadept.com/blog
parasiteblog.com

***

Merchandise

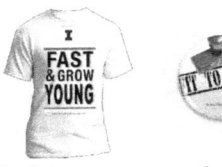

T-shirts, mugs, buttons
and more!

Tests & Quizzes

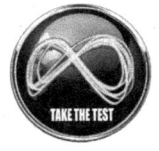 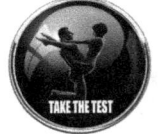

Longevity Test
Fit to Breed? Test

Available at www.agelessadept.com

Join the Ageless Adept Movement

*"Get exclusive healing protocols, behind-the-scenes
insight, and subscriber discounts on books & coaching."*

https://www.agelessadept.com/newsletter

The Power of the Paperback ▲

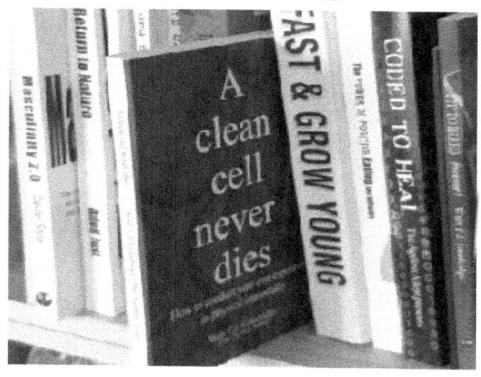

Digital books are convenient—but they're invisible, intangible, and easily forgotten. A paperback, on the other hand, has **mass, presence, and power**. It sits on your shelf, catches your eye, calls you back in, and keeps transmitting its wisdom long after you've turned the final page.

It whispers reminders, sparks curiosity in guests, and is far easier to share, gift, or revisit than a digital file lost in the cloud.

The paperback endures.

"A clean cell never dies" is more than just a title. It is a reminder as well as an optimistic ideal that is shared each time you or others glance at your shelf!

Order *https://www.agelessadept.com/shop*
***

Other Brands by the Author ▲

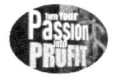 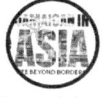 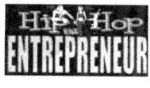 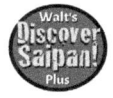

PassionProfit.com   JamaicaninAsia.com   HipHopEntrepreneur.com   DiscoverSaipan.com

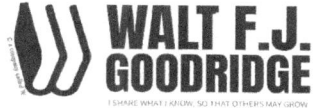

Or find them all at https://www.waltgoodridge.com